Rad Tech's Guide to
Mammography: Physics, Instrumentation, and Quality Control

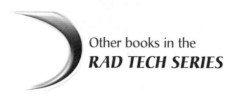

Other books in the
RAD TECH SERIES

Rad Tech's Guide to

Mammography: Physics, Instrumentation, and Quality Control

Donald R. Jacobson, PhD, DABMP
Assistant Adjunct Professor
Radiology and Biophysics
Medical College of Wisconsin
Milwaukee, Wisconsin

Series Editor
Euclid Seeram, RTR, BSc, MSc, FCAMRT
Medical Imaging Advanced Studies
British Columbia Institute of Technology
Burnaby, British Columbia, Canada

b
**Blackwell
Science**

©2002 by Blackwell Science, Inc.

EDITORIAL OFFICES:
Commerce Place, 350 Main Street, Malden, Massachusetts 02148, USA
Osney Mead, Oxford OX2 0EL, England
25 John Street, London WC1N 2BS, England
23 Ainslie Place, Edinburgh EH3 6AJ, Scotland
54 University Street, Carlton, Victoria 3053, Australia

OTHER EDITORIAL OFFICES:
Blackwell Wissenschafts-Verlag GmbH, Kurfürstendamm 57, 10707 Berlin, Germany
Blackwell Science KK, MG Kodenmacho Building, 7-10 Kodenmacho Nihombashi,
    Chuo-ku, Tokyo 104, Japan
Iowa State University Press, A Blackwell Science Company, 2121 S. State Avenue,
    Ames, Iowa 50014-8300, USA

DISTRIBUTORS:
The Americas
  Blackwell Publishing
  c/o AIDC
  P.O. Box 20
  50 Winter Sport Lane
  Williston, VT 05495-0020
  (Telephone orders: 800-216-2522;
      fax orders: 802-864-7626)
Australia
  Blackwell Science Pty, Ltd.
  54 University Street
  Carlton, Victoria 3053
  (Telephone orders: 03-9347-0300;
      fax orders: 03-9349-3016)

Outside The Americas and Australia
  Blackwell Science, Ltd.
  c/o Marston Book Services, Ltd.
  P.O. Box 269
  Abingdon
  Oxon OX14 4YN
  England
  (Telephone orders: 44-01235-465500;
      fax orders: 44-01235-465555)

Acquisitions: Beverly Copland
Development: Julia Casson
Production: GraphCom Corporation
Manufacturing: Lisa Flanagan
Marketing Manager: Toni Fournier
Cover and interior design: Dana Peick, GraphCom Corporation
Typesetting: GraphCom Corporation
Printed and bound by Western Press

Printed in the United States of America
01 02 03 04 5 4 3 2 1

Library of Congress Cataloging-in-Publication Data

Jacobson, Donald R.
    Rad tech's guide to mammography : physics, instrumentation, and quality
control / by Donald R. Jacobson.
        p. ; cm.—(Rad tech's guide series)
    title: Guide to mammography. Includes bibliographical references.
    ISBN 0-632-04499-3 (Pbk.)
    1. Breast—Radiography—Equipment and supplies. 2. Breast—Radiography—
Quality control. 3. Medical physics. 4. Radiography, Medical—Image quality.
    [DNLM: 1. Mammography—instrumentation. 2. Mammography—methods.
    3. Quality Control. WP 815 J17r 2001]
    I. Title: Guide to mammography. II. Title. III. Series.
RG493.5.R33 J33 2001
618.1'907572—dc21

2001001217

This book is dedicated to all mammography technologists. You all have such an important assignment. Please take good care of the special women in my life.

TABLE OF CONTENTS

SERIES EDITOR'S FOREWORD

Blackwell Science's Rad Tech Series in radiologic technology is intended to provide a clear and comprehensive coverage of a wide range of topics and prepare students to write their entry-to-practice registration examination. Additionally, this series can be used by working technologists to review essential and practical concepts and principles and to use them as tools to enhance their daily skills during the examination of patients in the radiology department.

The Rad Tech Series features short books covering the fundamental core curriculum topics for radiologic technologists at both the diploma and the specialty levels, as well as act as knowledge sources for continuing education as defined by the American Registry for Radiologic Technologists (ARRT).

The entry-to-practice series includes books on radiologic physics, equipment operation, patient care, radiographic technique, radiologic procedures, radiation protection, image production and evaluation, and quality control. This specialty series features books on computed tomography (CT)—physics and instrumentation, patient care and safety, and imaging procedures; mammography; and quality management in imaging sciences.

In *Rad Tech's Guide to Mammography: Physics, Instrumentation, and Quality Control,* Dr. Donald Jacobson, a renowned educator and expert in biophysics and radiology physics from the Medical College of Wisconsin, presents clear and concise coverage of the physics and instrumentation of mammography. Topics include fundamental physics of mammography, equipment components, image quality, and dose consideration, as well as quality control issues of primary significance to quality mammography.

Dr. Jacobson has done an excellent job in explaining significant concepts that are mandatory for the successful performance of quality mammography in clinical practice. Students, technologists, and educators alike will find this book a worthwhile addition to their libraries.

Enjoy the pages that follow; remember, your patients will benefit from your wisdom.

Euclid Seeram, RTR, BSc, MSc, FCAMRT
Series Editor
British Columbia, Canada

PREFACE

Rad Tech's Guide to Mammography: Physics, Instrumentation, and Quality Control is written from my teaching notes that pertain to the physics and technology of mammography. I have inflicted the pain that is usually associated with physics lectures in more than 100 mammography courses over the past 10 years. (Physics isn't really so bad.) *Rad Tech's Guide to Mammography: Physics, Instrumentation, and Quality Control* is designed to present information that will be helpful to those preparing for the mammography certification examination, as well as be a practical aid to those already performing mammography. Chapters 2 through 4 are ordered to correspond to the sequence of the steps involved in making a mammogram. Chapter 5 discusses image quality with reference to these same steps. Although not essential to the mission of this book, I have included small narratives in several places that should be of interest to the reader and will enhance the understanding of mammography. I often tell my students that physics is a way of looking at the world. Hopefully, *Rad Tech's Guide to Mammography: Physics, Instrumentation, and Quality Control* will help you deepen your understanding of the part of the world we call breast imaging.

Donald R. Jacobson

ACKNOWLEDGMENTS

I would like to thank Euclid Seeram, series editor, for inviting me to write this book. This is the first time that I have had to discipline myself to convert lecture material into a text. I am grateful for the support of my boss, Dr. Charles R. Wilson; my employer, the Radiology Department of the Medical College of Wisconsin; and Froedtert Memorial Lutheran Hospital for the opportunities that I have had to study mammography imaging. I very much appreciate the valuable assistance that I have received over the years from my clinical colleagues, especially Sally Molnar and Ann Gorman. Finally, I must thank my wife, Cathy, for 30 years of love and support.

—DRJ

CHAPTER 1

Why Mammography?

Breast cancer is an insidious disease that will affect one in eight women over their lifetime.[1] Although the probability is lower for younger women to contract breast cancer, approximately 20% of breast cancers occur in women in their 40s.[1] These cancers, if undetected, will cut the life of a person who is loved as a wife, mother, daughter, or friend tragically short. On the average, a women dying from breast cancer loses about 20 years of life.[1]

Each person began life as a single cell, a fertilized ovum, which began to divide. That cell became two, two became four, four became eight, and so on. Over a period of 9 months, that one cell multiplied into approximately 50 trillion cells, a baby. In an ironic twist of fate for some, one of these tens of trillions of cells, at some point in life, stops listening to its neighbors. This cell stops cooperating to support the organism and starts doing its own thing, becoming a rogue, and dividing uncontrollably. This rebel cell will become two, which will then become four, then eight, and continuing until, with approximately 100 million cells, it becomes a tumor that may be approximately 0.5 cm in diameter—a size that can be found with good mammography. In some cases, this transformation from a single cell into a lethal disease occurs in 6 months. In other cases, the tumor grows slowly over many years. The process of cancer induction and growth is not well understood. It is made more difficult by the fact that cancer is not a single disease; rather it is a spectrum of diseases.

The best prevention (mid-year 2000) is early detection. The best method for early detection of breast cancer is mammography, or as Dr. Bill Ecklund has said many times, "Not mammography, but *good* mammography." Figure 1-1 shows the progress that has been made in the last 40 years. Even when

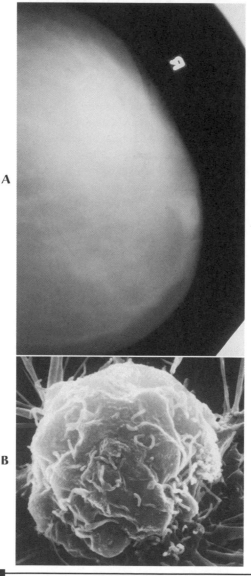

Figure 1-1 The challenge of breast cancer detection. *A,* This image shows where detection was 40 years ago. *B,* This image of a cancer cell represents where mammography technologists would like detection to be.

there is a 6 × 7 cm cancer in this breast, it is still difficult to visualize (see Figure 1-1, *A*). The image in Figure 1-1, *B*, from the National Cancer Institute is a single cancer cell and visualizes the stage at which detection may someday become a reality. Figure 1-2 demonstrates what good mammography looks like today. This patient presented with a 5 mm cancer in her left breast. Figure 1-2, *A*, is the mammogram and Figure 1-2, *B*, is the specimen radiograph of the cancer that was found and removed, freeing this woman from its ravage.

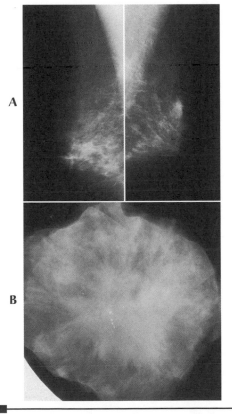

Figure 1-2 **The current state of mammography.** *A,* A 5 mm cancer that has been detected in screening mammography. *B,* The specimen radiograph is demonstrated.

Presently, early detection is the key to a good prognosis for the patient with breast cancer. Based on data supplied by the National Cancer Institute, 5-year survival for patients diagnosed with different stages of breast cancer are[1]:

- 96% for localized disease.
- 76% for regional disease (cancer has spread to axillary lymph nodes).
- 20% distant (cancer has metastasized)

All who are involved in mammography perform a critical task—a matter of life and death—and should do their best to do their best. After all, why provide mammography? Because people are important. As civilized beings, the infirmed among us are not discarded. The purpose of the money spent for and the great effort expended by the medical profession in general and by mammography in particular is for the purpose of extending, improving, or saving human life. To do their best, mammography technologists must master clinical, personal, and technical skills. The purpose of this book is to help them understand and, as a result, work best with the technical aspects of good mammography.

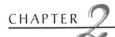

Mammographic Instrumentation and Physics

Chapter at a glance

INTRODUCTION

Producing quality mammograms involves five essential steps (Figure 2-1). These steps include the following:

1. X-ray production
2. X-ray absorption (including positioning the patient)
3. Recording transmitted x-rays
4. Processing the image
5. Viewing the image

The quality of the final image depends on the integrity of each step. This sequence is like the chain that is as strong as its weakest link. Optimizing image quality requires the optimizing each activity or process that contributes to the image. The better technologists understand the production of a mammogram, the better they can function as engineers of quality mammography and the better chance they will have to solve any problem that may arise.

Each of these five steps are considered. The relevant physics principles, instrumentation, and operation are explained. This material also provides the background for understanding image quality and quality control in Chapters 5 and 7, respectively.

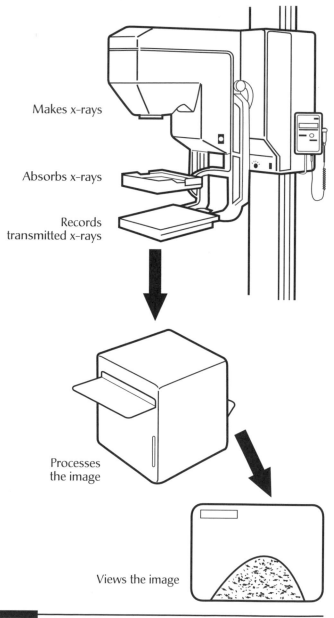

Makes x-rays

Absorbs x-rays

Records
transmitted x-rays

Processes
the image

Views the image

Figure 2-1 Five essential steps involved in the making of a
mammogram.

Instrumentation

The x-ray tube unit and the power supplies required to make it work (Figure 2-2) are considered first, with an emphasis on the features that are unique to mammography.

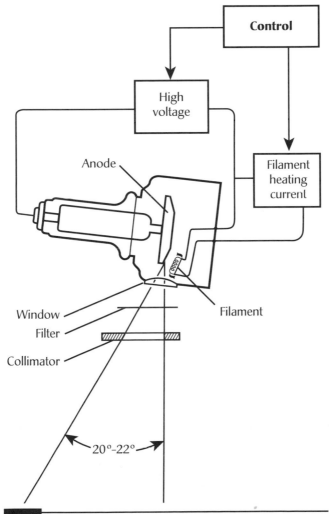

Figure 2-2 X-ray production is accomplished by the x-ray tube and associated power supplies.

Mammography X-Ray Tube, Filter, and Collimator

An x-ray tube is an example of an electronic device known as a diode because it contains two electrodes—the negative cathode and the positive anode. Electrons produced at the cathode are accelerated by high voltage to the anode where they interact to produce x-rays. The air has been pumped out of the tube (it contains a vacuum), thus the projectile electrons can travel all the way to the target with little chance of losing significant energy from bumping into air molecules. When they reach the target, the electrons typically are traveling at approximately half the speed of light (roughly 100,000 miles per second). An inside view of a modern mammography x-ray tube is shown in Figure 2-3.

Cathode. In most mammography tubes, the cathode contains two tungsten-thorium filaments, one for the large focal spot and one for the small focal spot. They operate *white hot*, similar to the headlights of a car. (If a person stares into headlights, then he or she will have a good idea of how the filament in an x-ray tube appears during an exposure.) The electrons that comprise the tube current (milliampere [mA]) are emitted thermionically. Some properties of the cathode are the following:

- The filament for the large focal spot (typically 0.3 mm) usually operates at a maximum of 100 mA tube current (some manufacturers offer higher current).

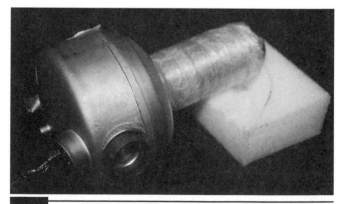

Figure 2-3 Inside an x-ray tube, the anode, focal track, filaments for large and small focal spots, and beryllium window are seen.

- Tube current is often reduced at high or low kilovolts peak (kVp).
  - ❏ High kVp from target-heating limitations
  - ❏ Low kVp from space-charge limitations
- The filament for the small focal spot (typically 0.1 mm) operates at 25 to 35 mA tube current.
- The cathode side of x-ray tube is always toward the patient.

The small focal spot sizes and consequent low tube currents of these tubes are dictated by the high spatial resolution requirements of mammography.

Anode. The positive electrode of the x-ray tube is the anode. The kinetic energy of the electrons is converted into x-ray energy in a thin layer of the incident surface of the anode, which is referred to as the target.

- All modern mammographic tubes have a rotating anode. With a typical anode diameter of three inches (7.6 cm), the area of the focal track is approximately 250 times larger than the area of the actual focal spot (see Figure 2-3).
- The typical anode heat capacity is 300,000 heat units (HU).
- The anode side of the x-ray tube is always located away from the patient.
- The material comprising most of a typical mammography anode is molybdenum (chemical symbol Mo).

Target material. The target of an x-ray tube is the surface of the anode that is bombarded by the electrons to make x-rays. Most of the material making up the anode of a general diagnostic x-ray tube is also molybdenum, but a thin layer of tungsten alloy serves as the target in these tubes. Some properties of mammography x-ray tube targets are as follows:

- For approximately 99% of mammography exposures made in this country, the target material is molybdenum. The reason for this choice will be examined later.
- Two manufacturers of mammography x-ray tubes offer a choice of target materials:
  - ❏ General Electric (Model DMR) offers molybdenum and rhodium (Rh).
  - ❏ Siemens (Model M3000) offers molybdenum and tungsten (W).

- Tungsten has a higher melting point and a higher atomic number, giving more efficient x-ray production.
- Molybdenum and rhodium have been chosen as mammography targets to take advantage of their characteristic radiation.

The characteristic x-ray energies are determined by the energy difference between electron orbits and are unique for every material. The x-ray energies of molybdenum and rhodium are in a range that is desirable for mammography. The effects of characteristic radiation is discussed later in thus chapter. Table 2-1 summarizes some properties of anode materials used in mammography.

Anode angle. Another unique feature of a mammography x-ray source is the anode angle (i.e., the angle between the surface of the target and a vertical line that is perpendicular to the image receptor). The anode angle has significant effects on image quality (Figure 2-4).

- *Anode heel effect:* The output decreases from its maximal value on the cathode side of the field, which is the chest wall, to the far anterior edge. An example of the resulting decrease in image optical density (OD) is shown in Figure 2-5.
- *Variable focal spot size (line focus principle):* The length of the projected or effective focal spot is greatest on the cathode side (chest wall) and decreases to zero at the anode cut-off in the far anterior field. This characteristic is demonstrated in the multiple pinhole picture of a typical mammography focal spot in Figure 2-6.

TABLE 2-1 **Typical Mammography X-Ray Tube Target Specifications**

TARGET MATERIAL	MOLYBDENUM	RHODIUM	TUNGSTEN
Chemical symbol	Mo	Rh	W
Melting point	2623° C	1964° C	3410° C
Characteristic energies (within the mammography range)	17.5 to 19.5 (keV)	20.5 to 22.5	none
Relative x-ray output	1	1.15	3

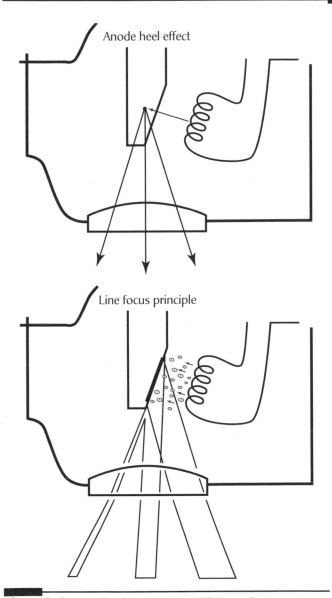

Anode heel effect

Line focus principle

Figure 2-4 The effects of the anode angle on radiation output include the anode heel effect and line focus principle. The radiation output and the focal spot length both decrease away from the chest wall.

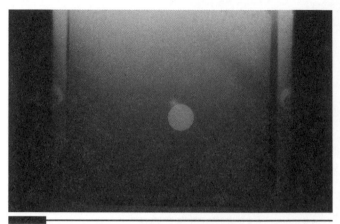

Figure 2-5 The anode heel effect is shown in this phantom image as a severe reduction in the optical density in the anterior aspect of the image.

Chest wall

Figure 2-6 The multiple pinhole picture of a mammography focal spot demonstrates the decrease of focal spot length moving from the chest wall to the anterior field. The distortion of the focal spot is demonstrated at the extreme edges of the x-ray field.

The anode angle determines the relationship between the actual focal spot on the target and the projected or effective focal spot, which is a factor in determining the spatial resolution of the image.

- A large anode angle produces a larger projected focal spot size (poor spatial resolution) and larger x-ray field size.
- A smaller anode angle results in a smaller projected focal spot size (better resolution) and smaller field coverage.

The following are some details regarding anode angles:

- A range of 6 to 13 degrees represents the anode angles for typical diagnostic x-ray tubes.
- From 20 to 22 degrees is a typical anode angle for a mammography x-ray tube. This angle is usually the sum of two angles (see Figure 2-2).
  - ❏ The angle of the anode within the tube is typically 16 degrees.
  - ❏ The tilt of the x-ray tube is typically 4 to 6 degrees.
  - ❏ One notable exception is the CGR (Compagnie Général de Radiologie, now General Electric Company) mammography x-ray tube, which has a unique design incorporating a 0 degree anode angle (for the large focal spots) and a 22 degree tube tilt.
- Some manufacturers provide a different anode angle for the large and small focal spot. The angle for the small focal spot is typically 9 to 10 degrees less than for the large focal spot, which has been accomplished in two ways:
  - ❏ A bi-angle tube has an anode with two different angles corresponding to the large and small focal spots.
  - ❏ In the GE-CGR mammography systems, the angle of the entire tube unit is changed when switching from large to small focal spots.
  - ❏ The small anode angle is always used with the small focal spot, and the larger anode angle is used with the large focal spot.

X-ray tube window. A window is needed that is strong enough to contain the vacuum in the x-ray tube while offering as little attenuation as possible to the low energy x-ray photons needed for mammography. In the early days of mammography, diagnostic x-ray tubes with glass windows were commonly used. However, the glass attenuated too much of the beam. The window used in modern mammography tubes has these characteristics:

- The material is *Beryllium*. Beryllium (atomic symbol Be) has an atomic number of only 4 and a density of 1.8, which are both the lowest for any metal.
- The thickness of the window is typically 0.8 to 1.0 mm.

X-ray filter. Filtration in an x-ray beam removes the low-energy photons that have no possibility of contributing to the image but would only contribute to patient dose, particularly skin dose. Severe skin burns have occurred during mammography exams when interlocks failed and a patient was irradiated with no added filtration in the x-ray beam. The total filtration in any diagnostic x-ray system, including mammography, must be greater than or equal to 0.5 mm *aluminum equivalent* to satisfy federal regulations. This does not mean that aluminum must be used as the filter; however, whatever material is used, its attenuation of the x-ray beam must be at least as much as 0.5 mm of aluminum would be. Filtration used in mammography imaging is described as follows:

- The material most commonly used as a mammography filter is molybdenum.
  - ❑ Typical thickness is 25 to 30 microns (0.025 to 0.030 mm).
  - ❑ Molybdenum or tungsten targets are used.
  - ❑ K-edge of absorption is 20,000 electron volts (20 kilo electron volts [keV]).
  - ❑ When a selection of filter materials is available, molybdenum is the best choice for 80% to 85% of patients in a typical screening program.
- An alternative x-ray beam filter commonly supplied on modern mammography imaging systems is *rhodium*.
  - ❑ A thickness of 30 microns (0.03 mm) is typical when used with molybdenum or rhodium targets.

❑ A thickness of 50 to 60 microns (0.05 to 0.06 mm) is typical when used with a tungsten target.

❑ K-edge of absorption is 23.2 keV.

❑ X-ray beam energy is *increased* with the use of a rhodium filter.

❑ Rhodium will be the most appropriate choice of filter for thick, dense breasts that comprise approximately 15% to 20% of a typical screening population.

■ An aluminum filter is provided by some manufacturers.

❑ A typical thickness is 0.5 mm.

❑ Aluminum k-edge of attenuation is far above the mammography energy range.

❑ Aluminum filtration is not considered appropriate for routine mammography because it results in an excessive energy x-ray beam for effective mammography imaging.

Molybdenum and rhodium, when used in mammography, are examples of a special class of filters referred to as *k-edge filters*. As in characteristic emission energies, the k-edge attenuation energy is also unique for all materials (it has exactly the binding energy of each of the two electrons in the K shell). At the k-edge energy for any material, the x-ray attenuation of that material increases abruptly (typically, approximately six times) with a corresponding drop in transmission. The effect on mammography x-ray beam energy and the reasoning for choosing these materials as filters will be explained later in this chapter.

Beam limitation (collimation). In the early days of mammography, the x-ray beam was limited to the breast being imaged using either movable blades or D-shaped diaphragms. The disadvantage of this type of collimation is that much of the film was clear, allowing the unattenuated bright light of the illuminator to shine into the radiologist's eyes. This situation will almost certainly interfere with film evaluation and diagnosis. Currently, the recommendation is to collimate the x-ray beam to the *film*. The reasons for the change in thinking are as follows:

■ The patient dose remains the same.

■ There is no increase in scattered radiation since the whole breast is irradiated in both cases.

■ The slight increase in scattered light (in the screen) is of no consequence to image quality.

■ A totally exposed film is *self-masking* (i.e., it acts as its own viewing mask, which significantly improves the visibility of subtle features on the film).

Accurate collimation is most critical at the chest wall side of the x-ray beam. The unique requirements for mammography are explained in Chapter 3.

X-Ray Generator

The mammography x-ray tube requires two power supplies, which together are often referred to as the x-ray generator.

■ *Filament heating power supply:* The filament temperature determines the number of electrons emitted thus the tube current (mA) and the quantity of x-rays. A hotter filament emits more electrons. Typical values are 10 volts and 5 amps (50 watts).

■ *High-voltage power supply:* The kVp determines the energy of the electrons bombarding the target and is therefore one of the factors, along with target and filter material, that subsequently determine the energy of the x-rays produced. The typical range for mammography is 22 to 32 kVp. Typical maximum power would be 35 kVp $\times$ 100 mA = 3500 watts (3.5 kW).

In the early days of mammography, single-phase (1Φ) and three-phase (3Φ) general diagnostic generators were used. These generators were undesirable because of the large voltage ripple they produce. The definition and values for voltage ripple are as follows:

$$\text{voltage ripple} = \frac{\text{maximum voltage} - \text{minimum voltage}}{\text{maximum voltage}} \times 100\%$$

WAVEFORM	VOLTAGE RIPPLE
1Φ (60 Hz)	100%
3Φ (6 pulse, 180 Hz)	~25%
High frequency (10 to 100 kHz)	~5%

When the kVp is changing during an exposure, the x-ray energy is also changing. Some important effects of the x-ray beam energy (which depends on the high-voltage waveform) are:

■ Radiation dose
■ Image contrast

- X-ray output rate (affects exposure time)
- Uniformity of target heating (has an effect on tube performance over the life of the tube and is better for a low-ripple high-voltage waveform)

Ideally, the high voltage would have a single constant value, corresponding to a ripple factor of zero. Modern mammography imaging systems employ high-frequency generator technology, which offers a reduced high-voltage ripple factor as one of its benefits.

High-Frequency Generator Technology

Mammography was actually one of the first applications of high-frequency x-ray generator technology when it was introduced in the mid 1980s. Now, it is commonly employed and will increasingly become the standard technology for energizing all x-ray tubes. Some benefits of high-frequency generator technology are as follows:

- Smaller and lighter generator (more compact)
- More constant output voltage (less voltage ripple)
- Repeatable and accurate x-ray technique delivery
- Closed-loop feedback
  - ❑ Generator monitors output voltage
  - ❑ *Feedback* from output to input of high-voltage transformer
  - ❑ Produces more constant output energy (kVp)
  - ❑ Filament heating current is also regulated by mA feedback, which produces a more consistent tube current (mA)

The following is a brief explanation of how the high-frequency generator works. It will help the reader understand the benefits that high-frequency technology offers to the practice of mammography (Figure 2-7).

- At the far left is the power source, where the unit is either plugged into an outlet or connected to a circuit breaker box. Single-phase power is almost always used with high-frequency generators.
- Inside the generator, the 60 Hz alternating current power is first converted to a direct current (flowing in one direction only). Ideally, this voltage would be constant, for example, 250 volts.
- This direct current is then fed into the inverter. As the name implies, the inverter flips the voltage from positive

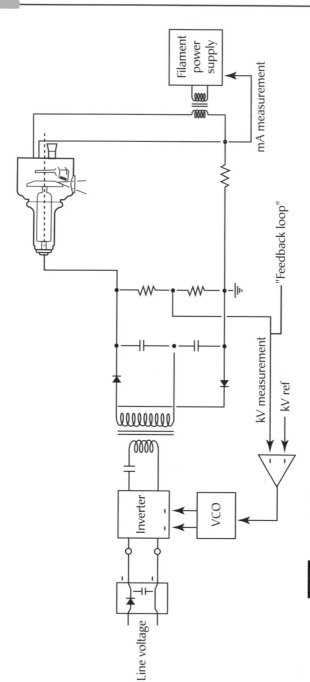

Figure 2-7 Simplified circuit diagram for a high-frequency generator. A major benefit to the practice of mammography is the accuracy and repeatability of x-ray techniques.

to negative, thus the positive 250 volts comes out of the inverter as a square wave that flips between positive and negative 250 volts. This changing voltage is required for the step-up, high-voltage transformer to work.

■ The step-up transformer produces an increase in the voltage, which, in combination with the two diodes and capacitors, produces an output voltage of, for example, 26,000 volts (26 kVp).

■ The positive voltage is connected to the anode and the negative to the cathode.

■ Every pulse that comes out of the inverter places a quantity of electrical charge on the output capacitors.

■ The capacitors store the charge and serve as a reservoir that helps keep the output voltage constant.

■ Because the inverter operates at high frequency, typically 10 to 100 kHz, the ripple of the high-voltage output is low, typically about 5%.

The real benefit of the high-frequency generator is the part of the circuit labeled as the *feedback loop*.

■ The feedback loop senses the output voltage through a pair of resistors connected across the output.

■ This actual measured voltage signal is compared with a reference signal by an electronic device known as a *comparator*.

■ If the kVp is right, then the measurement signal will be the same as the kV reference, and the output of the comparator will be zero. If the kVp is high, then the comparator will have a positive output, and if the kV measurement is low, then the comparator will have a negative output.

■ The output of the comparator is fed to the controller of the inverter, a circuit called a voltage-controlled oscillator (VCO).

Thus a continuous measurement of the output voltage is compared with a reference, with the difference being sent back to the input.

■ If the kVp suddenly drops during the exposure (as it may if the elevator next door starts to operate), then the kVp measurement would sense that change and feed back the message, "Give us more charge" to the inverter. After receiving this message, the inverter will increase the charge that it feeds into the high-voltage transformer, which returns the voltage to the value that it should be.

■ If the kVp has increased for any reason, then the feed-back loop would cause the inverter to decrease the charge fed into the high-voltage transformer to bring the kVp back to the desired value.

The net result of the feedback loop and its benefit is the following: *With a high frequency x-ray generator, more accurate and more repeatable x-ray techniques are the results.*

A feedback loop on the filament heating supply maintains a constant tube current (mA) and therefore a constant x-ray exposure output rate.

Physics of X-Ray Production and Attenuation

Characteristics of X-Rays

X-rays are exactly the same thing as visible light; that is, x-rays and visible light are both electromagnetic radiation, and both are waves that travel through space at 300 million meters per second and transfer energy from one point to another. Additionally, electromagnetic radiation occasionally behaves as though it was composed of tiny particles, which are called *photons*. The following points highlight the differences in the properties between visible light and x-rays:

■ Visible light has a wavelength of approximately 1 micron (10^{-6} m), which is roughly the size of a cell, with typical energy of 2 to 3 electron volts (eV).

■ Mammographic x-rays have a wavelength of approximately 0.1 nm (10^{-10} m), which is roughly the size of an atom. This dimension is often referred to as an Angstrom unit (Å). A typical energy for mammographic x-ray photons is 18,000 electron volts (18 keV).

Physics of X-Ray Production

Electromagnetic radiation is produced by moving electrons that are experiencing acceleration or that lose energy by changing energy states. In an x-ray tube, three essential processes occur to produce x-rays:

■ Electrons are produced at the cathode.

■ These electrons are accelerated to the anode by high voltage.

- The high-speed electrons from the cathode interact with the atoms in the target in one of three ways:
  - ❏ Approximately 99% of the interactions occur with outer shell electrons that produce heat, as well as visible and infrared radiation.
  - ❏ Of the other 1% of interactions that produce x-rays, about 20% to 30% occur with inner shell electrons to produce characteristic x-rays.[2]
  - ❏ The other 70% to 80% of the 1% of electron energy that is converted to x-ray output creates bremsstrahlung (a German term for *braking radiation*) by interacting with the nucleus of target atoms as follows:
    - The coulomb (electrical) attraction between the (−) electron and the (+) nucleus causes the electron to change direction, accelerating toward the nucleus.
    - This acceleration of the electron produces electromagnetic radiation, or in this case, an x-ray.
    - Close encounters, which are highly improbable, result in large acceleration and high-energy x-rays.
    - Weak interactions, when the electron is far away from the nucleus, are more probable and result in the production of low-energy x-rays.

Vignette

To understand why close encounters between projectile electrons and target nuclei are improbable and therefore why most bremsstrahlung x-rays have low energy, it is helpful to have a mental picture of how the target appears to the incoming electrons. Picture the following image in your mind. If we magnify the target atoms until their diameter, as defined by the outer electrons, is about the size of a basketball, then the spacing between atoms will also be about the size of a basketball. If we magnify the atoms until the nucleus is the size of a basketball, then the next nucleus will be approximately 10 miles away. If we picture the nucleus as basketballs, spaced 10 miles apart, the rarity of close encounters between the electrons (also about the size of basketballs in our mental picture) and nuclei indeed becomes easy to understand.

Mammographic x-ray output. All diagnostic x-ray beams, including mammography, contain a wide range of energies. The energy content of an x-ray beam can be described using the *x-ray energy spectrum*. Understanding this concept is important because image contrast and patient radiation dose both strongly depend on the x-ray energy spectrum. Again, there is usually a trade-off:

■ High x-ray energy produces relatively low contrast and low dose.

■ Low x-ray energy results in higher contrast with higher dose.

To illustrate this trade-off with x-ray energy, the following table shows the calculated contrast and required incident radiation exposure that results from imaging a 4.5 cm, 50-50 breast with x-rays of different energies (do not confuse keV with kVp). The contrast is expressed as the difference in optical density (OD) between a 0.5 cm tumor and surrounding adipose tissue.

X-RAY ENERGY	TRANSMISSION	REQUIRED EXPOSURE	IMAGE CONTRAST
30 keV	25%	40 mR	0.02 OD
25 keV	17%	60 mR	0.05 OD
20 keV	7.5%	133 mR	0.10 OD
15 keV	0.7%	1430 mR	0.32 OD

keV, Kilo electron volt; *mR*, milliroentgen; *OD*, optical density.

Note that over this energy range, there is a 30-fold increase in radiation dose to gain 15 times higher contrast. Tumors with a difference of less than 0.1 to 0.2 OD with respect to the surrounding tissue in a mammogram will almost certainly be undetected. This thought experiment demonstrates why mammography is performed at low energy. In the United States in the year 2000, decisions regarding the appropriate mammography x-ray technique were usually made based on the priority of improved detection over decreased dose. This concept is examined in greater detail in Chapter 6.

Mammography x-ray energy spectrum. When the complex shape of the mammography x-ray energy spectrum is understood, the reason molybdenum is usually chosen for the target and filter of the mammography x-ray source will also be understood. The x-ray energy spectrum is typically displayed using a graph. This graph, as is the case with a picture, is "worth a thousand words." To help understand the spectrum

(Figure 2-8), some explanatory terms have been added. The features of the mammography x-ray energy spectrum are as follows:

- The x-ray output below some arbitrary energy minimum (approximately 10 keV) is *none*. The purpose of the x-ray filter is to remove low-energy photons from the beam.
- Above this minimum, as the energy increases, the radiation output increases slowly.
- At 17.5 keV, the output shoots up to a high value (a lot).
- It then drops back to follow the normal gradual increase until it reaches 19.5 keV.
- At 19.5 keV, there is another sharp increase in output.

These two spikes of increased output occur at the characteristic x-ray energies for molybdenum and are the reason that molybdenum is chosen for the target in a mammography x-ray tube.

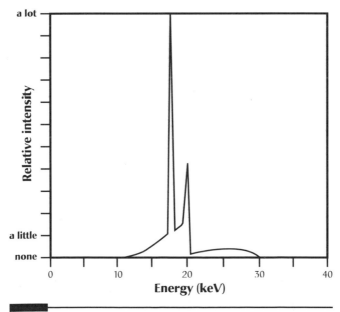

Figure 2-8 Typical x-ray energy spectrum for a mammography x-ray beam produced with a molybdenum target and molybdenum filter.

- Just above the second characteristic spike, there is a dramatic drop-off in the x-ray output, nearly down to *none*.
- As the energy increases further, there is a small increase in the output intensity, up to a maximal (albeit small) value.
- Above the energy corresponding to this output intensity maximum, the x-ray output again tapers off to *none* at the maximum energy.

What is the maximum energy in any x-ray beam, including mammography? The maximal energy is exactly equal to the kVp used to produce the exposure. Consider the following:

- High voltage (kVp) is the accelerating *force* that imparts kinetic energy to the electrons as they travel from the cathode to the anode.
- 30 kVp across the x-ray tube gives 30 keV of *energy* to the electrons striking the target. (An electron volt is the energy gained by one electron accelerated by one volt.)
- These electrons interact with the atoms of the target to produce x-ray photons having all energies up to (but not greater than) 30 keV.
- Increasing the kVp increases both the energy and the x-ray output.
  - ❏ The value of the maximum energy increases.
  - ❏ The total output intensity increases, including the 17.5 and 19.5 keV spikes.

As previously explained, the dramatic drop-off in output at 20 keV is due to the k-edge of attenuation for the molybdenum filter. K-edge filters are used in mammography for the following reasons:

- At the k-edge, the x-ray attenuation of a material abruptly increases (approximately sixfold), which means that the transmission through that material drops off dramatically.
- The use of a k-edge filter effectively reduces the quantity of higher energy photons in the mammography x-ray beam.
- Reduction in the number of high-energy photons is desirable because they would produce an image with lower contrast.

To summarize, *the net result of using a molybdenum target and molybdenum filter is the production of an x-ray beam that has a rel-*

atively narrow energy spectrum, with most of the output being in the range of 17.5 to 20.0 keV.

This energy range is optimal for imaging most patients undergoing mammography. However, imaging thick or dense breasts requires a more penetrating x-ray beam with higher energy, which can be accomplished quite effectively by replacing the molybdenum filter with a rhodium filter. Some considerations for switching to the rhodium filter are as follows:

- The k-edge of x-ray attenuation for rhodium is 23 keV (3 keV higher than molybdenum).
- The effect of replacing the molybdenum with the rhodium filter is to put x-ray photons between 20 and 23 keV back into the x-ray beam.
- This effect means that the rhodium filter gives a *higher* energy x-ray beam compared with molybdenum.
- The increase in energy from replacing the molybdenum with the rhodium filter is approximately the same as increasing the kVp by a factor of four. In other words, 24 kVp with a rhodium filter produces the same effective energy as 28 kVp with a molybdenum filter.

Alternative target materials. General Electric, with its model DMR mammography imaging system, also provides the choice of a rhodium target. This target is also used with the rhodium (or infrequently, the aluminum) filter.

- The rhodium target produces characteristic radiation that is 3 keV higher than molybdenum (approximately 20.5 and 22.5 keV).
- The combination of rhodium target and rhodium filter, Rh-Rh (at kVp values greater than 30) provides a further increase in x-ray beam energy compared with Mo-Mo or Mo-Rh.
- This higher energy beam is more penetrating and is the most appropriate choice for a small percentage of patients where it yields similar image quality for less radiation dose compared with a Mo-Mo or Mo-Rh exposure.[3]

Siemens model M3000 along with molybdenum also offers the choice of a tungsten target in combination with a molybdenum or rhodium filter. Rhodium-rhodium (at high kVp), tungsten-rhodium, and the use of the aluminum filter produce a higher energy x-ray beam, which is appropriate for patients with thick and dense breasts. These combinations serve only a small portion of the typical patient population.

Summary of Target–Filter Combinations
(listed in the order of increasing energy)

TARGET/FILTER	TYPICAL USAGE (this may vary)
Mo/Mo	80% to 85%
Mo/Rh	15% to 20%
Rh/Rh (above 30 kVp) or W/Rh	few %
Rh/Al	rare

Attenuation of X-Rays

The attenuation of an x-ray beam refers to the removal of photons from the beam as it passes through an object. During routine mammography, approximately 95% of the incident photons are attenuated by the breast. Attenuation of x-ray photons occurs by two mechanisms, *photoelectric absorption* and *Compton scatter.*

- With photoelectric absorption, the incoming x-ray photon is absorbed by an atom and delivers all of its energy to an inner electron, ejecting it from the atom.
  - ❏ The x-ray photon disappears, completely removed from the beam.
  - ❏ Photoelectric interactions are beneficial to x-ray imaging because they are the most important source of image contrast.
  - ❏ The ejected electron carries away most of the energy of the incident x-ray photon and is the primary agent for depositing energy for the patient, which is the patient radiation dose. (This process is discussed further in Chapter 6.)
  - ❏ The probability of photoelectric interaction increases with atomic number and decreases with energy, according to the following relationship:

$$\text{Probability of photoelectric interaction} \propto Z^3/E^3$$

  Where: Z is the atomic number of the absorber
  E is photon energy

  - ❏ Photoelectric interactions are dominant at low x-ray energies.

❏ Mammographic imaging technology and technique (target, filter, and kVp) are chosen to provide a low-energy x-ray beam to maximize photoelectric attenuation.
■ In Compton scatter, the incoming photon interacts with an atom and shares its energy with an outer-shell electron.
    ❏ The electron is ejected from the atom.
    ❏ The photon persists but with diminished energy, and its direction is changed.
    ❏ The scattered photon carries no information about the imaged breast and, if absorbed by the image receptor, it will actually decrease the contrast in the image.
    ❏ Probability depends on the electron (and therefore the tissue) density.
    ❏ Relatively independent of energy
    ❏ Dominates at higher energies
Overall x-ray attenuation depends on the following factors:
■ *X-ray beam energy, which depends on:*
    ❏ kVp
    ❏ Voltage waveform (ripple factor)
    ❏ Filter material and thickness
    ❏ Anode material
■ *Patient factors:*
    ❏ Breast thickness, which depends (within limits) on breast compression
    ❏ Breast tissue density and composition
■ *Other factors:*
    ❏ The compression paddle removes photons from the beam *before* breast exposure.
    ❏ The breast support, grid, and cassette cover remove approximately 50% of the primary photons from the beam *after* transmission through the breast.

Description of x-ray attenuation. The effective energy of any diagnostic x-ray beam, including mammography, is conveniently measured and described by performing multiple measurements of the attenuation of the beam. The thickness of a material required to cut the beam intensity in half is called the half-value layer (HVL) for that material.

■ Typical HVL of a mammography x-ray beam is 0.33 mm of aluminum.

- For soft tissue, the HVL is approximately 7 mm, which means that every 7 mm of tissue traversed by the beam reduces its intensity by one half.
- *Example:* A 4.2 cm breast is approximately 6 HVL (42 mm divided by 7 mm). Each HVL cuts the beam intensity in half, thus 6 HVLs transmit approximately 1.5%.
- This process is one definition of exponential attenuation and is illustrated for a 4.2 cm breast:

	# OF PHOTONS	TRANSMISSION (%)
Input: 1000		
Transmitted through:		
7 mm of tissue	500.0	50.0
14 cm of tissue	250.0	25.0
21 cm of tissue	125.0	12.5
28 cm of tissue	63.0	6.3
35 cm of tissue	31.0	3.1
42 cm of tissue	15.0	1.5
Output	**15.0**	**1.5**

This process is expressed mathematically as:

$$\text{Transmission} = (1/2)^N$$

Where: N is the number of HVLs traversed by the beam

In the example above:

$$(1/2)^6 = 0.015 = 1.5\%$$

Differential absorption. The difference in radiation absorption between tissues being imaged is often referred to as *differential absorption*. This quantity is important because of its significant contribution to image contrast. In mammography:

- The contrast of a tumor or calcification with surrounding normal breast tissue depends on the following factors:
  - The difference in atomic number (Z)
    - Z for all soft tissues is approximately 7
    - Z of calcium is 20
  - The difference in density
    - Density of fibroglandular tissues is approximately 1
    - Density of adipose tissue is approximately 0.93

- Density of calcifications (calcium apatite) is approximately 3
- Gland-to-adipose contrast is mainly a result of density difference since the atomic numbers are similar

■ Thickness or diameter of the tumor or calcification

■ Tissue-to-calcium contrast as a result of the differences in density and Z

■ Type of surrounding tissue for mass lesions
  - ❑ Low contrast with glandular tissue (they are almost isodense)
  - ❑ Higher contrast when surrounded by adipose tissue

■ Contrast is spoiled by scattered radiation

■ Visibility of calcifications is also affected by the image noise

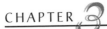
Performing the Examination: Technical Considerations

Chapter at a glance

INTRODUCTION

Now that the production and attenuation of x-rays have been considered, the performance of the examination (i.e., positioning the patient and making the x-ray exposure) is the emphasis. The geometry of mammography and other factors involved in performing the examination, including the patient, scattered radiation control, and technique factors, are examined.

GEOMETRY

Figure 3-1 shows the arrangement of the x-ray tube, collimator, compression paddle, breast support, grid, and film. Patient positioning and imaging geometry are two important aspects of setting up a mammography examination. Imaging geometry refers to the spatial relationship of the x-ray source, patient, and image

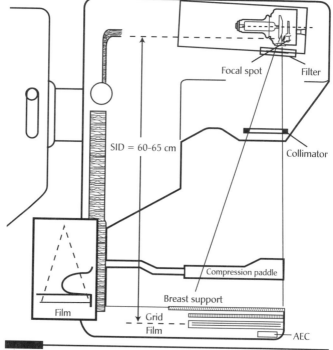

Figure 3-1 Typical geometry for mammography imaging system is demonstrated. Inset visualizes the important benefit of half-field geometry.

receptor. There are several unique aspects of mammographic imaging geometry as compared with general radiography:

- *Source-image distance (SID):*
  - ❑ 60 to 65 cm is typical.
  - ❑ Range is between 55 cm for some older units to 76 cm for one current manufacturer.
  - ❑ Some units offer variable SID (for example, GE-CGR model DMR SID can be 55, 60, or 65 cm).
- *SID effects:*
  - ❑ *Output intensity:* Inverse square law; longer SID means lower radiation exposure rate at the breast for a given output of the x-ray tube.

- ❏ *Magnification factor:* Larger SID gives lower magnification factor, thus a larger focal spot size can be tolerated.
- ❏ *Skin dose:* Shorter SID results in a higher skin dose for a given dose to the image receptor (from $1/r^2$ fall-off in radiation).
- ■ *Source-object distance (SOD):*
  - ❏ Equal to breast tissue thickness plus breast support-film distance (approximately 1 cm)
  - ❏ Greater for superior than inferior structures
  - ❏ SOD effects:
    - • Image magnification
    - • Skin dose
- ■ *Image magnification = SID/SOD (a trick to help remember:* SOD is on the bottom, like sod is on the ground)
  - ❏ Magnification increases as distance between the object and film increases.
  - ❏ A magnification of 1.0 (called contact mode) occurs only if the object is directly in contact with the film (SOD = 0) and for a zero thickness.
  - ❏ In mammography, 5% to 10% magnification (M = 1.05 − 1.10) is typical for standard (nonmagnification) imaging, often erroneously referred to as contact imaging.
  - ❏ In breast imaging, superior structures are imaged with higher magnification than inferior structures.

In what is usually referred to as *magnification mammography,* the breast is elevated about 12 inches (30 cm) above the image receptor. Consider the following facts:

- ■ The magnification factor will be typically between 1.5 and 2.0 for a magnification view.
- ■ For a magnification factor of 2.0, the object being imaged is halfway between the focal spot and film (refer to the previously mentioned definition and use either SID = 2 × SOD or SOD = $1/2$ × SID).
- ■ If the magnification platform is labeled M = 2, most of the breast is imaged at a magnification greater than two because of the thickness of the breast.
- ■ When performing a magnification view, a small focal spot must be used to decrease geometric unsharpness (formerly called the penumbra).

- The small focal spot requires a reduction in tube current to prevent damage to the target (typically 35 mA).

- A low mA means a longer exposure time. Exposure times can be as long as 6 seconds or even more for magnification mammography on some patients.

- For maximal image detail, there is an optimal magnification factor for every individual focal spot. Excessive magnification will make the image larger but not sharper.

- The magnification factor should be matched to the focal spot used. If there is a choice, experimentation by imaging the accreditation phantom at both magnification factors will determine which one gives the better image. (Using a magnifier, the imaged *detail* of the larger calcifications should be compared in the two images to select the optimal magnification factor.)

- A grid should not be used when performing magnification mammography. The Bucky mechanism should be removed or the cassette mounted in front of the grid. The air gap (distance) reduces the effect of scattered radiation on image quality (Chapter 3, page 40).

HALF-FIELD GEOMETRY

Half-field geometry is a unique but important feature of all modern mammography imaging systems (see Figure 3-1):

- The focal spot is directly above the chest wall edge of the breast support rather than being placed over the center of the anatomy to be imaged as it is typically for general radiography.

- The central ray of the x-ray beam is right *at the chest wall* of the patient and *parallel to it*.

- Half-field imaging is accomplished by moving the tube toward the patient and blocking the cathode half of the x-ray beam at the tube.

A diverging beam approaching the patient would exclude some tissue from being imaged (see Figure 3-1 inset). Because it is important to include all of the breast tissue in the mammogram, this divergence would be undesirable. Therefore effective mammography requires half-field geometry.

Disadvantages that coincide with half-field geometry include the following:

■ The anode angle must be large enough to cover the 24 cm width of the large image receptor for an SID equal to 60 to 65 cm (i.e., 20 to 22 degrees), which is twice the anode angle that would be required with conventional geometry.
■ The disadvantages of a large anode angle include the following:
  ❑ With a large anode angle, to produce the small projected focal spots required for mammography, the *actual* focal spot must be very small.
  ❑ The mA will thus be limited to prevent target damage.
  ❑ A low mA means longer exposure times.

Sometimes it appears as though radiology is just one big set of trade-offs.

PATIENT CONSIDERATIONS

The breast is difficult to image for the following reasons:

■ The inherent contrast is extremely low because breasts are composed entirely of soft tissue (fibroglandular and adipose).
■ There are no bones.
■ Contrast medium is not used (exceptions are the injection of air into a cyst after it has been aspirated and ductography).
■ Pathologic signs are subtle:
  ❑ Cancerous nodules have a density that is nearly identical to fibroglandular tissue. However, these nodules can be more easily visualized when they are surrounded by adipose, which has a lower attenuation. One of the advantages of compression in mammography is tissue spreading, which may move a nodule into an area of adipose where it can be detected.
  ❑ Microcalcifications produced by approximately one half of breast cancers have a high inherent contrast. These calcifications, however, are typically a fraction of a millimeter in size, and the resulting visibility in the image is diminished considerably.

A discussion of x-ray attenuation by breast tissues and subject contrast is presented in Chapter 5.

COMPRESSION

Compression of the breast is an important factor in the practice of optimal mammography. How much compression should be used? *As much as possible; but not too much.* Several important technical benefits of compression should be highlighted. These benefits include:

- Decreased breast thickness results in the following:
  - ❏ Lower radiation dose
  - ❏ Shorter exposure time
  - ❏ Less scattered radiation, which results in higher image contrast
- More uniform tissue thickness results in the following:
  - ❏ Smaller exposure range (also described as a narrow exposure latitude)
  - ❏ This narrower latitude allows the use of higher contrast film.
- Improved tissue structural visualization from tissue spreading
- Increased sharpness from decrease magnification factor
- Decreased potential for motion as a result of immobilization

Here are some important technical capabilities for breast compression that a modern mammography imaging system should have:

- Automatic and manual modes
- Foot-operated controls to free hands for positioning
- Adjustable initial compression force
- 25 to 45 pounds initial force applied (Mammography Quality Standards Act [MQSA] requirement after October 2002)
- Smooth, uniform application of compression force
- Compression paddle should be flat and parallel to the breast support (within 1 cm for all corners) to satisfy MQSA requirements
- Chest wall edge of paddle should be straight and parallel to the breast support

- There should be a wall on the paddle at the patient side to keep unwanted tissue and skin out of the image.
  - ❏ The wall should be parallel to the chest wall (perpendicular to the breast support) and have a smooth, rounded corner for patient comfort.
  - ❏ The compression paddle must not be visible in the image at the chest wall.
  - ❏ To meet MQSA requirements, the compression paddle must not extend more than 1% of the SID beyond the chest wall edge of the film.
- There must be a properly sized compression paddle for each film size.
- Compression should be maintained until released.
- There must be a manual release of compression in case of a power failure.
- Spot compression paddles should be available for both standard and magnification imaging.

SPECIFICATION OF BREAST COMPRESSION FORCE

Different measurement units are employed by various manufacturers to specify compression force. These units are as follows:

- *Newton (N):* Unit of force approximately equal to the gravitational force (weight) exerted on a mass of 100 grams (37 pennies have a combined mass of approximately 100 grams).
- Deca-Newton (dN) = 10 N
- One pound = 4.45 N = 0.44 dN
- 1 Newton = 0.22 pound = 0.1 dN
- 200 N = 20dN = (20 ÷ 0.44) = 45 lb
- 35 pounds = (35 × 4.45) = 156 N = 15.6 dN

BREAST SUPPORT

The breast support, which is located between the Bucky grid and the breast, supplies the lower component of the compression force. Desirable features are as follows:

- Low attenuation to transmitted x-ray beam
- *Sturdy:* The support must not bow under the compression force or encroach on the motion of the grid.

- *Carbon fiber is preferred:* When improperly manufactured, however, the carbon fiber pattern can be visible in the image.
- Smooth edges and a compact design to facilitate positioning for the mediolateral oblique (MLO) view

Automatic Exposure Control

Automatic exposure control (AEC) operates using a signal that is generated by an x-ray detector located behind the image receptor. The x-ray sensor should be positioned beneath the densest glandular tissue in the breast. The priority for proper x-ray exposure is adequate penetration of the glandular tissue since this is area where the radiologist will be looking for cancer. The detector must be highly sensitive since it receives only a small fraction of 1% of the x-ray exposure to the breast. Mammography exposure control has become sophisticated over the years. Some important features that are desirable in an AEC are:

- Multiple positions for the x-ray sensitive detector, at least in the posteroranterior direction (three to five positions is typical)
- Accurate markings on the compression paddle that correspond to the x-ray detector and that show the options for detector locations
- Lateral detector positions that are helpful for MLO and lateral views
- Smart sensors that derive information about the energy of the x-ray beam and that make corrections for the overall attenuation of the breast
- An AEC circuit that can terminate the exposure quickly when it senses that the back-up time will be reached. This feature prevents needless patient radiation dose for an exposure that would only have to be repeated.
- Accurate compensation for variations in breast thickness and kilovolts peak (kVp)
- Adjustable density control that gives a difference of approximately 0.15 optical density (OD) units per step
- A selection for multiple screen-film combinations is useful when image receptors with differing sensitivity are used or when there is a backup processor with a different speed than the main processor.

- Occasionally, compensation may be required to match the large to the small film sensitivity.

Some new mammography imaging systems offer multiple sensors that give the AEC the capability of automatically finding the detector that is closest to the densest glandular tissue and then using the signal from the detector (or combination of detectors) to time the exposure.

Full-Automatic versus Semi-Automatic Exposure Control

Most modern mammography imaging systems offer three choices of exposure modes. These choices with some considerations for their use are:

- *Full-AEC mode:*
  - ❑ In addition to automatically terminating the exposure, depending on the model, the imaging system will choose the values for some combination of kVp, filter, and target.
  - ❑ The choice of technique factors is based on patient and examination parameters that include breast thickness, tissue composition, and possibly, the measured x-ray attenuation of the breast.
  - ❑ One manufacturer (GE–CGR) makes a short x-ray preexposure to actually measure the breast transmission, and then during a short delay before the actual exposure, the technique factors are chosen.
  - ❑ The user may be given a choice of algorithms for selecting technique; for example, contrast, standard, or dose may be offered.
  - ❑ Another method is to change the kVp *on the fly* during the first few milliseconds of the exposure. The kVp is chosen to give an exposure time that will not exceed a maximal desired exposure time. The desired exposure time and range of kVp change (± 3 kVp is typical) is programmable by the installation engineer.
- *Semi-AEC mode:* Semiautomatic mode is the usual AEC function. The operator sets the x-ray technique (kVp, and possibly, filter and target materials) and initiates the exposure. The AEC terminates the exposure to produce the desired image optical density.
- *Manual mode:* In the manual mode, the technologist sets all exposure parameters, including kVp, filter, target,

and mAs. Manual mode is useful when AEC cannot operate properly, such as specimen radiography or imaging patients with breast implants.

All imaging systems with full AEC also offer semi-AEC and manual mode selection. When the full AEC mode is selected to image the patient, attention should be paid to the technique that is chosen by the computer. If the technologist disagrees with the selection, without hesitation, he or she should override the computer and select another technique and not *become just an "expose button pusher."*

Technique Charts

When mammography is routinely performed in the full AEC mode, a technique chart may seem superfluous. There are, however, reasons to maintain a technique chart:

- Consistency of AEC operation can be checked against a standard.
- Standardize the operation in multiple room facilities. Not all full AEC systems work the same, even when they are from the same manufacturer.
- Some technologists prefer to use semi-AEC mode.
- Specimen and implant imaging will usually require manual or semi-AEC operation.
- If the full AEC mode fails, then the technique chart can be used to maintain mammography service until repairs can be made.
- When there is no technique chart posted, MQSA regulations prohibit performance of mammography in the semi-AEC or manual mode in case of full AEC failure.

CONTROLLING SCATTERED RADIATION

Scattered radiation results from Compton interactions. The intensity of scattered radiation depends on the volume of tissue irradiated. In mammography, scattered radiation can be from approximately one half to more than twice the intensity of the primary beam. (The primary beam consists of photons that travel straight from the x-ray tube through the breast to the image receptor. These beams carry the information that is desired to record in the image.) Scattered radiation that is recorded on the image spoils image contrast and thereby reduces the diagnostic value of the exam. Reduction of scattered radiation is important and is accomplished in two ways.

Grids

A grid is built by aligning a series of thin attenuating strips (usually lead or tantalum) such that the primary radiation is passed through while most of the scattered radiation is attenuated (Figure 3-2, *A*). The spacers between the metal strips, required to hold them in place, are called the interspace material. Interspace material is a less attenuating material such as wood, plastic, or paper. Unfortunately, the material still attenuates the primary radiation. One exception is the HTC grid offered by LoRad Corporation. This grid has a honeycomb structure with open space (air) between the septa.

- The grid is positioned just underneath the breast support and above the film cassette.
- The grid should be a moving grid (Bucky mechanism).
- A useful grid descriptor is the *grid ratio,* which is equal to the height of the strips divided by the distance between them, written as:

$$\text{ratio (R)} = h/d$$

Where: h is the height of the strips
d is the separation between the strips

- A typical grid ratio for mammography grids is 4:1 or 5:1. This ratio is considerably lower than regular diagnostic grids (R = 8 − 12). Because of the low x-ray energies used, the grids must be thin (meaning that the h is small) to prevent excessive loss of primary radiation.
- The frequency of attenuating strips for mammography grids is typically 150 to 200 lines/inch (60 to 80 lines/cm).
- Carbon-fiber covers are preferred for their low attenuation.
- A mammography grid typically attenuates:
  - About one half of the primary radiation
  - Approximately 70% to 80% of the scattered radiation
- A grid improves image contrast but with a cost of increased dose.

The ratio of image contrast with a grid to the ratio without a grid is termed the *contrast improvement factor* (CIF). For mam-

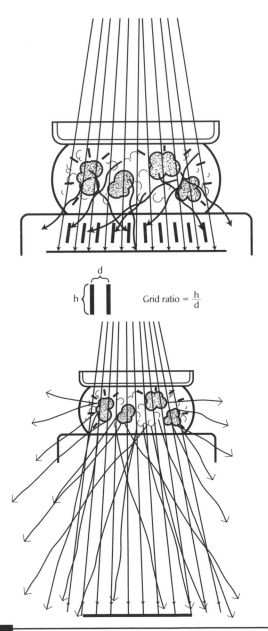

Figure 3-2 A grid or air gap is used to reduce the effect of scattered radiation in mammography imaging.

mography, typical improvement is 15% to 50%, depending on the grid effectiveness and breast thickness (CIF = 1.15 to 1.50).

Because both scattered and primary radiation is removed from the beam by the grid, the required x-ray exposure to produce a given optical density in the image increases. The ratio of required exposure with the grid to the ratio without the grid is commonly referred to as the *Bucky factor.*

Typical Bucky factors for mammography grids are 2 to 3. This value means that using a grid increases the patient dose by a factor of 2 to 3 compared with no grid.

Air Gap

Magnification is used in mammography to improve visualization of calcifications or other small, medium- to high-contrast structures. In magnification mammography, the breast is moved approximately 12 inches (30 cm) *away* from the film and *closer* to the x-ray source. The following are considerations for the use of this operating mode:

- Because the breast is moved closer to the x-ray source, the irradiated tissue receives a higher radiation dose compared with standard mode imaging.
- Example: If the magnification factor is two, then the SOD is cut in half, and the dose increase, calculated with the $1/r^2$ rule, is four.
- To compensate for this potential increase in radiation dose, the image receptor should be positioned in front of the Bucky grid or the Bucky mechanism should be removed for magnification mammography. Removing the Bucky cuts the required exposure by two or three times.
- The grid can be removed because the *distance* of the air gap separates the source of scattered radiation (the breast) from the image receptor thereby reducing the contribution of scattered radiation to the image.
- A clamp to hold the cassette or an open cassette holder is better than a closed tunnel, which attenuates 25% to 30% of the primary radiation.

Image Recording, Film Processing, and Image Viewing

Chapter at a glance

INTRODUCTION

The pattern of x-rays transmitted through the breast contains information on the anatomy and possibly the pathologic condition of the breast tissue. The next priority in the making of a mammogram is to record the transmitted x-rays (i.e., to capture the highest quantity of information in the image for transfer to the radiologist). As discussed in the previous chapter, the desire is to record *primary* radiation only, thus a grid or air gap is used to reduce the contribution of scattered radiation to the image.

IMAGE RECORDING

Direct Film Mammography

In the early days of mammography, the film itself was used as the detector. Direct film mammography required an unacceptably high radiation dose. There is no doubt that if this study were still performed using film alone, then there would be no screening mammography programs for women of any age. To understand why the required dose is so high, consider the following description of film and its performance as an x-ray detector (Figure 4-1):

- Film base is a polyester sheet approximately $8/1000$ of an inch thick (see Figure 4-1, part c).
- There is a gelatinous layer on both sides of the film.
  - ❑ The gelatin, which is the same as the gelatin that is eaten, is manufactured from animal skins.
  - ❑ A single gel layer would curl the film in the developer.
- The back gel layer (see Figure 4-1, part *b*) contains an antireflective dye (purple). Light reflected from the back of the film to the emulsion would spoil image detail.
- The front layer (see Figure 4-1, part *d*) holds the photographic emulsion (silver-halide crystals).
  - ❑ The light-sensitive layer on the film (emulsion) is only approximately $1/4$ of $1/1000$ of an inch thick.
  - ❑ This layer contains a mix of silver bromide (AgBr) and silver iodide (AgI), typically 98% to 99% silver bromide.
  - ❑ The film is notched. In the landscape orientation, the notch will be in the upper left or lower right corner when the emulsion is toward the operator.
- Native emulsion is sensitive to blue and ultraviolet light.
- Dyes are added to the emulsion to make the film sensitive to the green light emitted from mammography screens (known as *orthochromatic* films).
- The single-emulsion gel is thicker than double-emulsion layers.
- Single emulsions have as much silver as dual emulsions combined.
  - ❑ Therefore the single emulsion is *thicker* than the double emulsion.
  - ❑ *Usually* the single emulsion cannot be optimally processed with standard processing.
  - ❑ Most single-emulsion films have improved performance when processed with extended processing (see "Extended Processing" in this chapter).
- The film emulsion is not a good absorber of x-rays.

■ Approximately 99% of the x-ray energy passes through the emulsion.

Because most of the photons pass directly through the film emulsion, a large quantity of x-ray exposure, approximately *1 Roentgen* (R), is required to produce an image using film alone as the image receptor. (For more information on radiation units of measurement, see Chapter 6.) If 1 R is the required exposure to the film, then the patient exposure will be many Roentgens, a highly undesirable situation. However, when the film is placed into a cassette with an intensifying screen, the required exposure is approximately *100 times* less than when the film is used alone.

Screen-Film Image Receptors

The intensifying screen absorbs and converts x-ray energy into visible or ultraviolet light (see Figure 4-1). The following are noted:

■ A single-screen and single-emulsion film is used for maximal spatial resolution (image detail).

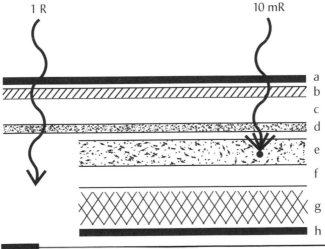

Figure 4-1 Early mammography was accomplished with direct film imaging. A cross section of a film and mammography screen/cassette image receptor is shown. Parts a and h are front and back covers of the cassette. Refer to the text fro more information.

- Film is placed in front of the screen with the emulsion facing the screen. A thin sponge (see Figure 4-1, part *g*) provides pressure.

- Modern mammography screens contain a rare earth phosphor (see Figure 4-1, part *e*) applied to a polyester base (see Figure 4-1, part *f*):
    - Gadolinium-oxy-sulfide (Gd_2O_2S:Tb) is standard.
    - (Gd_2O_2S:Tb) emits green light.

- The screen has high x-ray absorption efficiency (approximately 50% to 60%).

- Many light photons are emitted for each x-ray photon absorbed (an x-ray photon with 20 keV can potentially produce up to approximately 8700 green light photons with 2.3 keV each).

- An intensifying screen greatly increases the efficiency of the image receptor.

- Requires approximately 1% to 2% of the radiation needed to expose film alone.

- Spectral (color) matching between screen and film is critical, therefore orthochromatic film (dyes added) must be used.

Why is the screen located *behind* the film?

- Low-energy x-ray photons are absorbed by the screen within a short distance (i.e., near the front of the screen) to produce a small point of light called a *scintillation*.

- The size of the light spot (scintillation) enlarges as it spreads from the point of x-ray absorption.

- Thus the film emulsion is placed against front of screen, as close as possible to the point of x-ray energy absorption and subsequent light production.

- Intimate contact between the screen and film is critical (Figure 4-2, *A*).

If the requirement to have intimate contact between the film emulsion and screen is understood, then the mammographic technologist can also understand the importance of good film-screen contact. When there is a slight separation between the screen and the film (even $^1/_{1000}$ of an inch), the light from the x-ray scintillation will spread considerably, resulting in a loss of detail in the image (Figure 4-2, *B*). For this reason, the Mammography Quality Standards Act (MQSA) and the

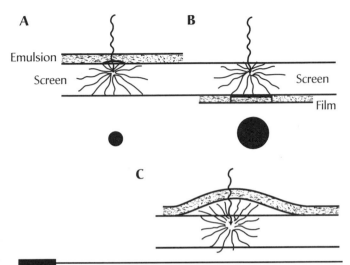

Figure 4-2 The film emulsion is placed directly in front of the intensifying screen to improve the detail of mammography imaging (A). Placing the film behind the screen (B) or any loss of contact between the screen and the emulsion (C) results in a loss of image detail.

American College of Radiology (ACR) requires that cassettes be tested semiannually for film-screen contact.

Screen-Film Cassette

Some characteristics and desirable features of the cassette are:

- Low x-ray absorption from front cover:
  - Absorption is approximately 30% for plastic cassettes.
  - Absorption is approximately 15% for carbon-fiber cassettes.
- Light tight
- Rugged
- Good film-to-screen contact is designed to *squeegee out* any trapped air
- Ability to place film edge as close to chest wall as possible
- Minimal effects of aging:
  - Screen output decreases
  - Screen may develop stains that cause artifacts
  - Screen-film contact may deteriorate

- New cassettes will likely be different than used ones.
- Care and cleaning are important. Follow the manufacturer's instructions.

Because trapped air can spoil screen-film contact and reduce image sharpness, it is important that mammography cassettes are allowed to *rest* as long as possible (10 to 15 minutes is recommended) before they are used after film loading. When possible, cassettes should be used in order (i.e., cassettes loaded first should be used first). A system should be implemented to place freshly loaded cassettes at the *back* or *bottom* of the stack.

Image Processing

After recording the transmitted x-ray exposure, the next step in the production of a mammogram is processing the film. Once exposed, the film contains what is referred to as a latent image. The latent image is composed of latent image centers (LIC), which are silver-bromide grains in the emulsion that have been hit by light. When the film goes through the developer, the LIC (crystals) are converted to metallic silver, which remain in the emulsion to produce the gray, dark, and black areas of the image. The process begins with the x-ray exposure and finishes in the developer. To obtain a visible image, the unimaginably small quantity of energy that is delivered by the x-ray photons is amplified a billion times, passing through the developer in the film processor.

Vignette

To understand the incredibly tiny quantity of energy required to produce a mammogram, consider the following thought experiment. You have a cup of coffee that has cooled to room temperature. If you, as I do, prefer your coffee hot, then you could place the cup in the microwave oven for a minute to heat the coffee. What would happen if you tried to heat the cup of coffee using x-ray exposures? Suppose you place the cup of coffee on the breast support and use a fairly high technique, for example, 35 kVp at 300 mA to deposit 1 rad of dose into the coffee for each exposure. How many exposures would be required to heat the coffee (assuming that you have a perfectly insulating cup that retains all the energy put into the coffee)? You will be surprised at the answer. Heating the coffee requires approximately 2,000,000 exposures. Another way of expressing this concept is that the exposure time would be approximately 2 months!

Film Processors

A typical hardware configuration for a mammography film processor is diagrammed in Figure 4-3. A film processor commonly used for mammography is demonstrated in Figure 4-4.

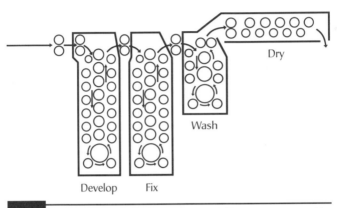

Dry

Wash

Develop   Fix

Figure 4-3 Schematic diagram of a typical film processor used in screen-film mammography imaging.

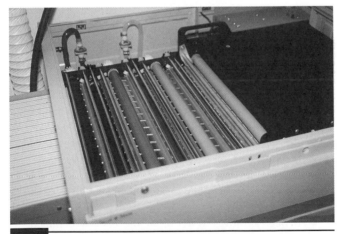

Figure 4-4 Commonly used processor for mammography imaging. Feed tray, input rollers, developer-to-fixer crossover, fixer-to-wash crossover, and film dryer are visualized *(from left to right)*. The two flexible hoses bring replenishment chemistry into the developer and fixer tanks.

An elaborate transport system incorporating over 100 rollers moves the film successively through three chemical tanks where it interacts with the chemistry that transforms the latent image into a visible image. Essential features, listed in order of film movement, include:

- Input tray
- Input rollers that sense when film is entering processor
- Deflector (with guide shoes) to direct film into the developer tank
- Developer tank and rack
- Developer-to-fixer crossover assembly with guide shoes
- Fixer tank and rack
- Fixer-to-wash crossover assembly with guide shoes
- Wash tank and rack
- Deflector moves film into the dryer where hot air blows over the film.
- Most rollers are one inch in diameter and made of rubber, hard or soft plastic, and phenolic or metal.
- The turn-around rollers in the bottom of the tanks are typically 2-inch rollers.

Film Processing

The interaction of the film emulsion, the developer, and the fixer in the processor is a chemical reaction. All chemical reactions depend on three variables—time, temperature, and chemical strength. To obtain optimal and consistent performance from the processor, these three variables must be kept constant. The operation of an automatic film processor is outlined in the following four essential steps of film processing:

- *Developing:* Exposed crystals (LIC) are changed to silver metal
- *Fixing:* Unexposed crystals are washed out of the film
- *Washing:* Removes any residual developer, fixer, or unexposed crystals
- *Drying:* Removes water from the emulsion, making it hard and tough

These steps will now be explained in turn.

Developing

- Determines speed and contrast of the image (the most critical step)

- Swells the gel containing the emulsion thus chemicals can penetrate
- Converts exposed crystals to metallic silver, which remains on the film to form the image
  - When silver-bromide molecules are broken apart to free the silver, bromide ions are released into the developer.
    - Developer with a proper bromide level is defined as *seasoned*.
    - When the processor is cleaned and the tanks are filled with new chemistry; *starter,* which contains bromide ions, is added to the new developer to give it *instant seasoning*.
- Produces chemical reaction (developer is *oxidized* and emulsion is *reduced*)
- Developer chemistry is complex
  - Contains roughly a dozen components.
  - All components must be present with sufficient quantity and freshness.
- All chemical reactions depend on three factors:
  - Time of development (measured from the moment the leading edge of the film enters the developer until it enters the fixer)
  - Temperature of the developer chemistry
  - Strength of the developer chemistry

Consistent processing performance requires constant control of the variables as previously listed. The following subsystems of the film processor are designed to provide this control:

- Mechanical subsystem (motor, gears, belts, and chains) determines the speed of film transport and thus controls the development time.
  - 24 seconds is typical in 90-second processing
  - 33 seconds is typical for a $2^{1}/_{2}$-minute processor cycle
- Recirculation subsystem (pump, heat exchanger, and filter) circulates the developer chemistry through a heat exchanger that senses its temperature and heats or cools it thus maintaining the desired temperature.
- A filter in the recirculation system removes contaminants from the developer.

- Replenishment subsystem (pump and replenishment source) adds fresh developer chemistry for each film processed to replace the developer that will be oxidized by that film thus maintaining a constant strength of the developer.
  - ❏ For proper operation, replenishment chemicals must be properly mixed and fresh. Follow the manufacturer's recommendations, but 2 weeks is typically the recommended maximal storage time.
  - ❏ To minimize oxidation, replenishment tanks should have floating lids to protect the chemicals from oxygen in the air.

In the developer, the silver bromide in the film emulsion is reduced and the developer chemistry is oxidized. Oxidized developer is inactive and useless for further film processing. (Severely oxidized developer is brown and must be discarded.) A small quantity of developer chemistry is oxidized (poisoned) by every film that is run through the processor, which is why effective and consistent replenishment is necessary.

Fixing

- Stops development process
- Removes unexposed silver crystals (produces clear areas on film)
- Shrinks gel, which squeezes out some of the water
- Has temperature control and replenishment systems

The silver bromide crystals that were unexposed to light are washed out of the film emulsion in the fixer, which is why silver collection is performed on the overflow from the fixer tank.

Washing

- Re-swells emulsion gel
- Removes all chemical residue

It is especially important to wash out any unexposed silver. Residual fixer-silver complexes that remain will cause the film to darken with time, and eventually the film will be unreadable. For this reason, tests are performed to measure the residual fixer (the fixer-silver complexes are the greatest concern).

Drying

- Removes retained moisture from emulsion gel
- Hardens gel further
- Allows dry film to be easily handled when it drops
- Set at the lowest temperature to produce dry films

Wet films are usually a sign of chemical problems and usually should not be corrected by increasing the dryer temperature.

Film Feeding and Chemistry Replenishment

How should films be run through the processor? In all processors commonly used for mammography, the input rollers sense the incoming film and activate the replenishment pumps while the film is entering the processor. The orientation and configuration of film entering the processor is important. Consider the following:

- Running with the emulsion up or down is neither right nor wrong.
  - Processor performance, film density, and contrast are usually not affected by the orientation of the emulsion.
  - Emulsion up means that the emulsion is running on the *inner* rollers, while emulsion down puts the emulsion in contact with the *outer* rollers.
  - Follow the film manufacturer's recommendation.
  - The technologist can experiment and determine for which orientation produces the cleanest film with the least noticeable artifacts.
- Films that run on the long and short side into the processor provide different replenishment.
- When two small films are run together (i.e., side-by-side), the replenishment rate must be doubled.
- It is important to know how the processor has been set up for replenishment; all technologists should follow the same procedure, which is generally the following:
  - Small films (18 × 24 cm) are run two at a time, side-by-side, with the short side parallel to the rollers.
  - Large films (24 × 30 cm) are run one at a time, with the long side parallel to the rollers.
- A minimal number of films must be run each day to have consistent processing performance.
- The minimal number of films required will vary with each film manufacturer, but it is typically between 30 and 60.
- When the film volume is low, less than the minimum, *flooded replenishment* is recommended to maintain the chemical strength.

❏ Flooded replenishment turns on the pumps at regular intervals, independent of the number of films that are processed.

❏ Rates will vary with manufacturer, but 65 cc of developer chemistry every 5 minutes is a representative flooded-replenishment rate.

❏ Running mammography films through a nondedicated processor (with other film types) is usually preferable to trying to maintain consistency using a dedicated processor with a low or inconsistent film volume.

Extended Processing

Extended processing in mammography is accomplished with higher developer temperature, longer development time, or both. Extended processing of most single-emulsion films results in higher speed (which means lower radiation dose) and higher image contrast. Some of the newer films, the Kodak M-2000 film in particular, are not recommended for use with extended processing. Note the following characteristics of extended processing:

■ *Increased development time:* 24 or 32 seconds is increased to 45 or 47 seconds, respectively.

■ *Increased total cycle time:* 90 and 150 seconds is increased to 180 and 210 seconds, respectively, as a result of increased development time.

■ *Increased developer temperature:* 92° F is increased to 95° F.

■ *Increased time and temperature.*

■ *Changing the developer temperature is inconvenient* in practice, because it may take 20 minutes to stabilize.

■ *Other required changes with extended processing:*
   ❏ Increased replenishment rates
   ❏ Decreased dryer temperature

■ *Effects on imaging* (for most single-emulsion films):
   ❏ Increased speed (lowers radiation dose by as much as 50%)
   ❏ Increased contrast (narrower latitude)
   ❏ Increased image noise resulting from lower dose (see "Image Noise" in Chapter 5)

Screen-Film-Processor Performance

The performance of a film processor or screen-film-processor combination is typically reported using the H & D curve, also referred to as a D-log-E, sensitometric, or characteristic curve (Figure 4-5).

H & D, D-log-E, or characteristic curve

- Film optical density (OD) graphed against sensitometer light exposure.

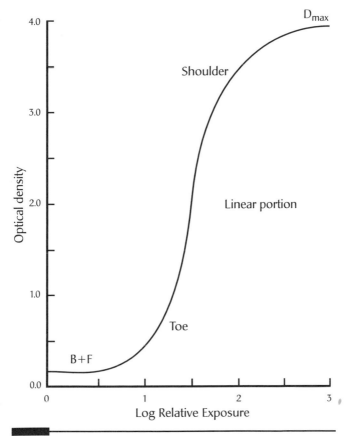

Figure 4-5 Typical H & D curve.

- ❑ The sensitometer gives the film a constant and reproducible light exposure, usually modified with a stepped optical attenuator.
- ❑ In the 21-step wedge, each two steps doubles the light exposure.
- ❑ Each step is 44% different compared with adjacent steps.
- ❑ The correct color exposure, blue or green, should be used to match the film sensitivity (always green for commonly used mammography films).
- ❑ Neither light output matches the screen output color spectrum exactly.
- ■ OD can also be graphed against radiation input exposure to characterize the screen-film-processor combination.
- ■ Features of the curve (see Figure 4.5):
  - ❑ *Base + fog (B + F), where there has been no exposure:* Minimal film density is typically less than or equal to 0.20 OD.
  - ❑ *Toe:* Region in which OD begins to increase with increasing exposure.
  - ❑ *Linear or straight-line portion:* Contrast is maximum where film should be used.
  - ❑ *Shoulder:* Region in which the slope of the curve (contrast) is decreasing.
  - ❑ *Maximum density (D_{max}):* Typically 3.5 to 4.0 OD for mammography film.

Descriptors of screen-film-processor performance include speed, contrast, and latitude.

Speed

- ■ Exposure required to produce a specified OD (typically 1.0 above B + F).
- ■ Speed is expressed in reciprocal Roentgens (1/R)
- ■ Typical mammography screen-film-processor system requires 10 milliroentgens (mR) exposure for a density of 1.2 (1.0 above the B + F), which corresponds to a speed of $1/0.01R = 100 1/R$, commonly specified as simply 100
- ■ Medium density (MD):
  - ❑ Processor control measurement that is related to speed
  - ❑ Sensitometer step with a density closest to 1.2

Contrast

- Contrast is the difference in OD for a given difference in exposure.
- The slope of the H & D curve is a measure of contrast.
  - ❏ High gradient (slope) indicates high contrast.
  - ❏ Contrast is highest in the middle part or the linear portion of the curve.
  - ❏ In the toe and shoulder of the curve, contrast is reduced.
- Contrast is expressed as:
  - ❏ *Gamma (γ):* Slope of the H & D curve at a point, occasionally specified at a given OD or at the slope maximum.
  - ❏ *Average gradient:* Slope between two specified densities, typically between 0.25 and 2.00 above B + F.
  - ❏ If B + F = 0.20, then the average gradient would be the slope between 0.45 and 2.20 OD.
- *Density difference (DD):* Processor control measurement, OD difference between two sensitometer steps, is typically:
  - ❏ The step with OD closest to but greater than 0.45
  - ❏ The step closest to 2.2 OD

Latitude

- Latitude is the range of exposure that gives OD values that lie within a desired range; for example, not less than 1.0 or greater than 2.5 OD.
- Too much contrast results in narrow latitude.
  - ❏ Glandular tissue may be imaged near the toe of the curve.
  - ❏ Low gradient (shallow slope) in the toe results in low image contrast.

OD of all glandular tissue in a mammogram should be greater than 0.8 OD. *A low-density mammogram is a low-contrast mammogram.*

Vignette

Two images produced on a patient several years ago demonstrate the trade-off of contrast and latitude (Figure 4-6). The left image was a result of the technique that was automatically chosen by the imaging unit. The right image was from the technologist overriding the automatic mode and choosing another low-energy technique. When the radiologist was asked about her preference, she immediately selected the right image, saying, "I like the higher tissue contrast here." However, after looking at the pair of images a little longer, it became apparent that the pectoral muscle is better penetrated in the left image where the lymph nodes are clearly seen. There is no information through the pectoral muscle in the right image. After a few minutes, the radiologist said that she wanted the parenchymal contrast of the right and the axillary contrast of the right. Of course, that is not possible.

The trade-offs are as follows:

- *Speed and detail:*
  - ❏ Spatial resolution is dependent on dominant silver grain (crystal) size in emulsion.
  - ❏ Small grains yield high detail but low speed (required dose is higher).
  - ❏ Large grain size yields less detail but requires less radiation exposure.
- *Contrast and latitude* (Figure 4-6):
  - ❏ Both are dependent on range of grain sizes in emulsion.
  - ❏ Small range in sizes give high contrast and narrow latitude.
  - ❏ Larger variety of grain sizes responds to a wider range of exposure levels (wide latitude) but yields lower image contrast.

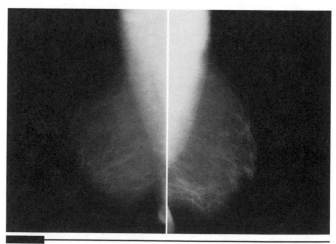

Figure 4-6 Image contrast and latitude are a trade-off. The image either has a high contrast but narrow latitude *(right)* or a wider latitude but lower contrast *(left)*.

Reciprocity failure. Film reciprocity refers to obtaining a constant OD for the same overall exposure, independent of exposure time or intensity. Reciprocity failure refers to the fact that for either extremely short exposures or extremely long exposures, the efficiency of film is reduced and more exposure is required to produce the same OD.

■ Exposure reciprocity usually holds in general diagnostic imaging; the same (intensity × time) *product* gives same OD.

■ Reciprocity failure occurs in mammography for the long exposure times often required, especially for magnification imaging.

■ For example, with modern commercial films, a 4-second exposure requires 25% to 50% more radiation to produce an OD of 1.5 when compared with the exposure required for an exposure of $^1/_{10}$ of a second.

Film reciprocity compensation is usually accomplished in the generator calibrations by the service person who installs or repairs the imaging equipment. Remember, as the exposure time increases, the dose required will also increase.

Film Data Sheet

The film manufacturer can provide data sheets for the film that a facility is using. It is advisable to obtain a copy and study these data sheets to determine the following properties:

■ Speed in 1/R
■ MTF (maximum lp/mm resolution)
■ Contrast or average gradient
■ Spectral (color) sensitivity
■ Performance improvement with extended processing:
  ❏ Increased developer temperature
  ❏ Longer exposure time

IMAGE VIEWING

Even when every other step in the production of a mammogram is correctly performed, and even when all available information has been collected on the film, it is still possible to overlook a cancer or signs of a cancer on the image if the image is not interpreted under optimal viewing conditions.

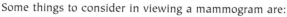

Some things to consider in viewing a mammogram are:

- *Illuminator:*
  - ❏ High-brightness film trans-illumination is required.
    - Necessary because mammograms are exposed to a higher OD than other diagnostic films.
    - Typical mammogram OD is in the range of 1.4 to 1.8 as compared with general radiographs, which are typically 1.0 to 1.2.
  - ❏ Uniform brightness and color is recommended for any bank of illuminators used to read mammograms.
  - ❏ Surfaces should be clean and free of dirt and marks, especially the diffuser plates behind the films (illuminators should be cleaned inside and out routinely).
  - ❏ Dedicated mammography viewers are best; mammography films cannot be read optimally on a general radiographic viewer.
- *Ambient conditions:*
  - ❏ Subdued, overhead lighting is best; not total darkness, but rather, a low-light level.
  - ❏ There should be no glare or reflections from the reading surfaces.
  - ❏ There should be no bright light sources behind the radiologist when films are read (such as a window or another film illuminator).
- *Other requirements:*
  - ❏ Bright light source or *hot light:*
    - Information is in the image at densities above what can be seen, even with a dedicated mammography film illuminator.
    - Information about skin line, nipple profile, and adipose tissue can be recovered.
    - Except possibly for some of the new composite-emulsion films, typically, the skin line and nipple profile should not be visible under standard viewing conditions.
    - Ideally, the bright light will be equipped with an iris to vary the size of the light field.

- ❏ 2× magnifier:
  - Doubles the size of the image on the retina.
  - Necessary because mammographic screen-film systems can resolve 20 line pairs per mm (20 lp/mm, 25 micron detail), which is beyond what the human visual system can see at a normal viewing distance.
- ❏ Masking:
  - Absolutely necessary for optimal viewing of mammograms
  - Greatly increases low-contrast detectability
- ■ *Any unattenuated light from the illuminator compromises mammography viewing.*

The improvement in the visualization of subtle details in a mammogram when it is properly masked is dramatic. If the facility has chosen to use the small diaphragm or collimator with *spot compression views*, then a mask that fits the image should be cut out of a large black film and used whenever these small format images are viewed.

The viewing conditions at the processor where the films are evaluated for quality should also be optimal and should match the diagnostic viewing conditions as closely as possible, including:

- ■ Illuminator brightness and color
- ■ Ambient lighting
- ■ Available accessories (at least a *hot light* and magnifier)

Because mammograms are exposed to a higher OD, a brighter light source is required to view the mammogram. The American College of Radiology recommends an illumination intensity that is equal to or greater than 3000 candles per meter squared (cd/m^2). A physicist should be able to help evaluate the illuminators if there is a question about their adequacy for mammography.

CHAPTER 5

Mammographic Image Quality

Chapter at a glance

INTRODUCTION

Any consideration of image quality in mammography must contain the basic purpose of the exam, which is to answer the question, "Does this patient have breast cancer?" Image quality requirements for mammography must be related to the task of diagnosing occult breast cancer. For this reason, all of us working in mammography need an understanding of both clinical and technical aspects of mammographic image quality.

The goal of optimized mammography is early and accurate detection of breast cancer.

IMAGING PERFORMANCE DESCRIPTORS

The accuracy of cancer detection has two components: sensitivity and specificity. Both components are important; one cannot be considered without the other. Speaking generally, there is a trade-off between the two aspects. Optimized mammography will provide some balance between high sensitivity and high specificity. This chapter begins with the definition of terms.

Sensitivity

The *sensitivity* of a diagnostic test can be described as how often a disease is detected when it is present. Sensitivity can also be described as the true positive fraction, which is the ratio of positive calls to the actual number of cancers. Another way of stating this concept is, "When cancer is present, how often is it found?" The general consensus is that the sensitivity of quality screening mammography is quite good, approximately 90%.

Specificity

The *specificity* of a diagnostic test is how often, when the diagnosis is positive, that the disease is actually present. Specificity can also be related to the true negative fraction (ratio of true negative calls to [true negative + false positive] calls), which will be 100% when the number of false positive calls is zero. Another way of stating this is, "When the diagnosis is positive, how often is that diagnosis correct?" The specificity of screening mammography is not good. Studies have reported between 50% and 80% specificity, which means that many women undergoing surgical biopsies do not have cancer.

To illustrate the trade-off:

- If all cases are called positive, then the sensitivity is 100%, but the specificity is poor (unless every patient has cancer).
- If all cases are called negative with no false positive diagnoses, the specificity is 100%, but there are also no true positives (i.e., all cancers are missed).

CLINICAL IMAGE QUALITY REQUIREMENTS

What are the pathognomonic signs of cancer on a mammogram? What does the radiologist see in the image that allows her or him to make a diagnosis of cancer? The following section is not meant to be a lesson on mammographic interpretation; rather, it is a physicist's understanding of a few of the important mammographic manifestations of cancer, based on many interactions with clinical colleagues. Three important findings are listed that, when present on a mammogram, can lead to a diagnosis of cancer.

High-Density Mass

A mass that has high density, compared with adipose, can be benign or malignant. (The high tissue density results in the mass having a *lower* optical density [OD] in the image.) The features of the mass, in particular, its shape and the characteristics of its margin provide clues that allow differentiation of benign and malignant masses.

- A benign mass will typically present the following characteristics:
  - Round or oval shape
  - Smooth, well-demarcated, and completely visualized margin
  - Sharply defined border sometimes surrounded by a halo
- Most common benign breast masses are fibroadenomas and cysts.
- Indications suggesting malignancy include the following:
  - Irregular or lobulated shape or both
  - Indistinct, fuzzy, or nonvisualized margin
  - Indentations in the margin (occasionally referred to as the *tent sign*).
  - Spiculations, spokes, or tentacle-like radiations extending from the mass

The spiculations associated with breast cancer are likely a result of an enzyme imbalance caused by the cancer that travels out along fibrous tissue planes to produce the classic spoked or spiked appearance.

Vignette

Based on a retrospective study of several hundred of his mammography reports, Dr. Peter Dempsy found that the words *spiculated mass* in the diagnosis were the most reliable indicators of breast cancer.

Microcalcifications

Approximately 50% of the cancers detected with mammography produce calcifications. This number of cancer cases is important, however, because the cancers detected by microcalcifications are usually less advanced. As with masses, breast calcifications can be either benign or malignant. The characteristics of benign calcifications are similar to characteristics for benign masses, including the following:

- Round, smooth shape
- Well-defined
- Occasionally a lucent center

Common causes of benign calcifications are:

- Mastitis
- *Milk of calcium:* Milk of calcium is dissolved calcium in the fluid within the acini at the terminus of the milk ducts and can be diagnosed by comparing the craniocaudal (CC) view with the lateral view. In the CC view, the calcifications will be round and in the lateral view, they will have a *teacup* appearance.

Calcifications caused by cancer are a result of the death of cells lining the terminal ducts. The dying cells spew their contents, including calcium, into the duct. The shape and distribution of calcifications can provide important indicators about their origin:

- Linear patterns of calcification and linear branching patterns of calcification can be indicative of cancer.
  - ❑ When the linear or branching patterns are solid, referred to as *rodlike,* the calcification could be a result of calcified ducts caused by secretory disease, another benign condition.
  - ❑ When the linear or branched linear structures resemble a dotted line, the probability of cancer increases.
- The shape of malignant calcifications in a mammogram has been described as *crushed stone* or *broken needle tip*.
- Another term often used to describe a cluster of malignant calcifications is *pleomorphic*, designating a variety of sizes and shapes.

Architectural Distortion

Skin dimpling or nipple retraction can be described as advanced architectural distortion. However, long before these features are visible externally, the normal parenchymal architecture will likely be disturbed by the disease process. Technologists who have performed a great deal of mammography have learned to recognize the typical parenchymal patterns of normal breast tissue. Features that do not follow the expected pattern may provide important clues that will aid in finding a subtle cancer. For example:

- A concave instead of convex trajectory
- Straight or linear structure, appearing stretched
- A radiating pattern resembling spokes in a wheel

These mammographic manifestations of cancer are all clearly illustrated in the specimen radiograph of a breast cancer shown in Figure 5-1.

TECHNICAL DESCRIPTORS OF IMAGE QUALITY FOR MAMMOGRAPHY

From this point on, the discussion of image quality focuses on the technical aspects of image quality, specifically:

1. Spatial resolution
2. Image contrast

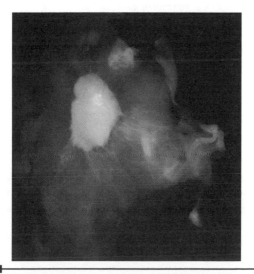

Figure 5-1 Specimen radiograph of a breast cancer demonstrating many of the common classic features of malignancy in a mammogram.

3. Optical density
4. Image noise
5. Image artifacts

The technical factors that affect each component of image quality is outlined. These pages are designed to assist in maintaining or optimizing image quality and to present an easy-to-follow outline showing the relationship between technical factors and image quality in mammography.

Spatial Resolution

Spatial resolution refers to the ability of an imaging system to separate small objects that are close together. Related to and referred to as image detail, spatial resolution is usually measured with a lead or gold foil, line-pair pattern or multiple bar pattern. Mammography imaging systems are capable of resolving 20 lp/mm.

Vignette

Spatial resolution is often reported in line pairs per mm (lp/mm). To convert lp/mm into the size of imaged detail, use the following procedure: twenty line pairs indicate 20 lines and 20 spaces of equal size. The imaged detail can be equated to the size of a resolved line. Because there are a total of 40 lines and spaces in a millimeter, each line and space is 1/40 mm (0.025 mm) or 25 microns.

- *Effective focal spot size:*
  - ❏ Actual focal spot size
  - ❏ Anode angle
  - ❏ Position in x-ray field (anteroposteriorly [AP] and laterally)
  - ❏ Shape of focal spot
- *Geometry and magnification factor:*
  - ❏ Magnification = SID ÷ SOD. The magnification for standard mode is typically 1.05 to 1.10; in the magnification mode, the magnification is typically between 1.5 and 2.0.
  - ❏ Magnification imaging requires the use of the small focal spot to minimize geometric unsharpness (penumbra).

- ❑ Object-film distance (OFD) is equal to the source-image distance minus the source-object distance. A larger OFD corresponds to higher magnification.
- ❑ Breast thickness is a factor in magnification. Thicker breasts and breast features located superior are imaged with higher magnification than the breast's inferior structures in the CC view.
- ❑ Compressing the breast moves tissues closer to the film, reducing magnification factor and, in most cases, improving spatial resolution.
- ❑ Support film distance is the spacing between the inferior breast tissues and film (CC view), typically 1 cm.

Motion is a common problem in mammography. A prominent mammographic technologist has stated that she sees some effects of motion in almost every mammogram that she reads. The factors that contribute to the probability of motion in a mammogram include:

- ■ *Exposure time:*
    - ❑ kVp and required mA
    - ❑ Milliroentgens (mR)/mA or the output of the x-ray tube; varies from manufacturer to manufacturer, and occasionally, from tube to tube.
    - ❑ Breast thickness and composition; thicker and denser breasts require more exposure thus a longer exposure time.
    - ❑ The exposure time required to produce a high OD is obviously longer than what would be required to produce a low OD mammogram. However, accepting a low OD mammogram for any reason is a poor choice, as will be demonstrated later.
    - ❑ A compressed breast is a thinner breast and requires less exposure thus a shorter exposure time.

The most effective way to shorten exposure time in mammography is to increase the kVp. Increasing the kVp, even by one-half, can result in an effectively shorter exposure time. Increasing kVp has two beneficial effects:

- ■ As the kVp is increased, the radiation output for a given mA increases.

- Higher kVp provides higher efficiency of x-ray production (mR/mAs).
- At higher kVp, the energy is higher thus making the beam more penetrating.

Note that the automatic exposure control (AEC) density compensation is *not* included in this list. When the OD of a mammogram is low, especially when it is a long exposure time, changing the density compensation to +1 or +2 will result in only a longer exposure time and the situation will become worse. Because of reciprocity failure, a longer exposure time will require a higher radiation dose.

- *Screen-film combination:*
  - ❑ Mammography x-ray film has an intrinsic spatial resolution of hundreds of lp/mm.
  - ❑ The limiting component in the image receptor is the x-ray screen.
  - ❑ Because mammography screens are thin and only one is used, the screen-film image receptor is capable of high spatial resolution (20 lp/mm).
- *Magnification mammography:* Because the object is enlarged on the image receptor, the resolution within the object is improved when the small focal spot is used.
- *Screen-film contact:* As explained in Chapter 3, the slightest air gap between the screen and film can result in a significant loss of spatial resolution. Cassette design and integrity is important to maintain intimate film-screen contact.
- *Viewing the image:* A magnifying lens is required to view mammograms because the human visual system is not capable of resolving details that can be recorded with modern film-screen imaging systems (20 lp/mm). The magnifying lens, typically 2× magnification, enlarges the image on the retina of the eye, which allows the visual perception of all of the detail recorded in the mammogram.

Spatial resolution, or detail, in a mammogram is important. Visualization of calcifications and fine fibrous structures, as well as clear demarcation of the margins of masses is important in breast cancer detection. Perception of a solitary micro-calcification is not strictly dependent on spatial resolution alone. This task is often described as high-contrast detectability. High-contrast detectability depends on both spatial resolution and image noise, which is discussed later in this chapter.

Image Contrast

- *Subject contrast:* Defined in this text to include both the energy of the x-ray beam and the tissue contrast presented by the breast being imaged.
  - ❑ *Breast composition:* Contrast in a mammogram results from the difference, albeit small, between glandular and adipose tissue. Some breasts do not contain enough glandular tissue to produce a high-contrast mammogram. It may not be possible to image a 1 cm or 2 cm, fatty-replaced breast with high contrast because the tissue contrast is not there. (Going to a low kVp, such as 22 or 23 kVp, will help in these cases, as is discussed later in this chapter.)
  - ❑ *Calcium:* Calcium produces higher contrast. However, calcifications are small, and therefore other factors such as spatial resolution and image noise contribute to their visibility in the image.
  - ❑ *Effective x-ray beam energy:* The following factors contribute to x-ray beam energy (see Chapter 2). High energy generally means low contrast and vice versa.
    - KVp
    - Voltage ripple factor
    - Filter material and thickness: The standard filter material is molybdenum. Switching to a rhodium filter results in a higher energy x-ray beam.
    - Target material: If offered on an imaging system, rhodium (above 30 kVp) or tungsten targets will result in a higher energy x-ray beam.
- *Scattered radiation:* Scattered radiation is to contrast what motion is to spatial resolution (i.e., scattered radiation spoils image contrast). Scattered radiation is detrimental to image quality; therefore a grid or air gap is used to

reduce its effect, although a penalty of an increased radiation dose is paid. The following factors pertain to scattered radiation:

- ❑ *X-ray beam energy:* The production of scattered radiation is slightly greater for higher energies but is not a major factor in mammography.
- ❑ *Volume of tissue irradiated:* The larger the quantity of tissue that is irradiated by x-rays, the more scattered radiation is produced. The volume of tissue irradiated depends on two factors:
  - *Radiation field size:* Spot collimation results in less scattered radiation (to maintain a given full-field OD, the mA for a small spot view should be increased, usually by approximately 10%).
  - *Breast size and composition:* Breast compression results in less effect from scatter because the scattered radiation is spread over a larger area. Improved contrast is one of several benefits of breast compression.

■ Effectiveness of methods is used to reduce the contribution of scattered radiation to the image.
  - ❑ Grid
  - ❑ Air gap

For a discussion of the effectiveness of grids and air gaps in removing scattered radiation from the transmitted beam, see Chapter 3.

■ Image receptor
  - ❑ *Screen*
  - ❑ *Film:* The film is the dominant component in the image receptor for image contrast. As discussed in Chapter 4, the mix of silver grain sizes in the emulsion of the film determines the inherent contrast of the film.
    - *Film fog:* Fogging of film is an overall increase in the OD that has a similar negative effect on image contrast as that caused by scattered radiation. The base plus fog (B + F) OD of the clear area of any mammography film should not exceed 0.20. Possible causes of film fog are:
    - *Age of the film:* It is important to establish good habits in the use of mammography film when it arrives at the facility.

- *Film usage:* Usage should be according to *FIFO* (i.e., first in, first out). Always use the oldest film first, which can be easily accomplished by placing new shipments of film behind the boxes currently in stock. (Film should be stored in a vertical orientation.) Using film in the order it was received has two important benefits: (1) the oldest film is used first, and (2) film emulsion batches are used sequentially.

- *Storage conditions:* It is possible to contribute to film fog by improper storage conditions, which may include temperature, humidity, and chemical environment. All manufacturers have recommendations for the limits of temperature and humidity when film is stored. Typical numbers, and an easy sequence to remember, are *30-50-70* (i.e., 30% to 50% relative humidity and 50° to 70° F). These recommendations may not be exact for all manufacturers, but they will be similar.

- *Darkroom conditions:* Darkroom problems include light leaks, defective safe light filter, light bulbs above recommended wattage, and x-rays entering the darkroom. Detecting darkroom fog and light leaks are required quality control tests.

- *Chemical fogging:* The darkroom may not be a good place to stock new film because of the potential for processor chemistry (especially the developer) to be in the air. When there is a question, it is recommended that the film supplier be consulted.

❏ *Film processing:* Although film processing has no direct effect on spatial resolution, it is important in the production of image contrast. The important parameters of film processing that effect image contrast are developer temperature, development time, and developer strength.

❏ OD is a factor that does not always appear in a list of the determinants of image contrast. However, OD is important and is perhaps the most neglected aspect of mammography image quality (see Figure 4-5).

As the density level decreases, approaching the toe of the curve, the contrast (slope) decreases. A low OD mammogram is a low contrast mammogram. It is better to increase the kVp to get adequate tissue penetration than to produce a light film at lower kVp (Figure 5-2). An OD of 0.8 is suggested as the minimum acceptable OD in any area of the mammogram, especially in the dense glandular tissue. *A densitometer should be used if there is a question.*

- *Masking:* Image masking is essential for optimal viewing of mammograms. Although masking an image does not change the contrast of the film, it dramatically improves the visible or perceived contrast as that film is evaluated.
- *Unattenuated bright light:* Any light from the illuminator severely compromises the viewing of a mammogram.

Image Optical Density

As discussed in the previous section, the OD of a mammogram is important. The higher optical densities to which mammo-

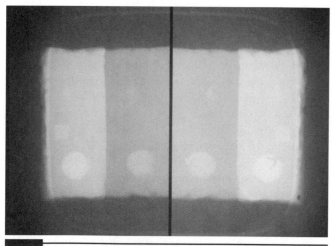

Figure 5-2 A low OD mammogram is a low–contrast mammo-gram. This tissue–equivalent phantom demonstrates the benefit of adequate tissue penetration. The image on the left, which was produced at 30 kVp, has 20% higher contrast than the image on the right, which was produces at 24 kVp. The higher contrast is the result of the better penetration and higher OD of the higher kVp image (1.25 OD), compared with the lower kVp image with a background density of 0.75 OD.

grams are exposed result in higher image contrast because moving up on the H & D curve results in a higher gradient (steeper slope) (Figure 5-3) (see Figure 4-5).

The considerations for image OD are:

- Radiation exposure or radiation output
  - ❏ kVp
  - ❏ mA
  - ❏ AEC: controls the delivered mAs
  - ❏ Anode material
  - ❏ Filter
  - ❏ SID
- *Patient:* The fraction of the x-rays incident on the breast that is transmitted depends on the following:
  - ❏ *Breast thickness*
  - ❏ *Compression:* A compressed breast is a thinner breast and the transmission is increased.
  - ❏ *Breast tissue density:* Glandular tissue is more attenuating and transmits less x-ray exposure than adipose tissue.
  - ❏ *Scattered radiation to film*

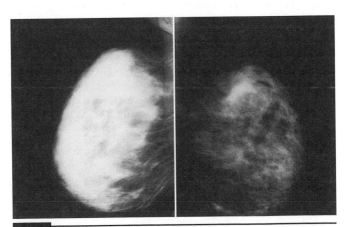

Figure 5-3 Which image is underexposed? Both are. Although the overall exposure of the film on the right was considered optimum, the small island of glandular tissue has an 0.6 OD. Microcalcifications will not be seen in glandular tissue imaged at a low OD as a result of image contrast. This study would benefit from a spot view of the underpenetrated glandular tissue.

Although scattered radiation contributes to the image OD, it reduces contrast, thus every attempt should be made to reduce its contribution to the final image. When scattered radiation is removed from the x-ray beam, increased radiation exposure is required to achieve a given OD. The contribution of scattered radiation to the image depends on the following factors:

- Quality of scattered radiation produced
  - X-ray beam energy
  - Volume of tissue irradiated
- Effectiveness of scatter clean-up
  - Grid
  - Air gap
- Image receptor

The screen was the primary contributor to spatial resolution in the image and film was the dominant component for image contrast. The overall efficiency of the image receptor depends on both the screen and the film. Using film that is designated to be compatible with the screens that are being used is extremely important. One particular detail that should be known is whether the screen and film are chromatically (color) matched. When there are questions about compatibility, the film manufacturer should be consulted first.

- *Film processing:* As with contrast, developer temperature, strength, and time directly affect the density of a film after exposure.
- *Viewer intensity:* The intensity of illumination of the viewbox or film changer, although it does not change the actual OD of the film, it will affect the apparent or the perceived film density.
- Because of the higher OD to which mammograms are exposed, bright view boxes are strongly recommended.
- The recommendation of the American College of Radiology is that the illumination source be greater than 3000 candela per meter squared (cd/m^2). Luminous intensity has also been reported in *nits*, but cd/m^2 is the preferred unit.
- Mammograms, which are read on standard, nondedicated illuminators should appear overexposed.

- For the darker areas of a mammogram, which may still include useful information, a bright source or *hot light* is a required accessory, which should usually include the assessment of skin line and nipple profile.

Image Noise

Image noise is perhaps least understood and the aspect of image quality for which technicians have the least comfort. Brief consideration of acoustic noise will help us to understand image (visual) noise and its effect on image quality. Acoustic noise can be described as static or as any unwanted sound that interferes with the communication of information.

Vignette

Suppose that you are going to take a trip, and as you leave town, you tune in your favorite radio station. As you travel away from your home, the signal becomes weaker and more static is heard. Eventually, the signal will be so weak or the static so strong that you may be tempted to turn up the volume. If you have ever done this, then you realize that increasing the volume only makes the situation worse; the dominant noise just becomes louder. In frustration, you will eventually change the station or turn the radio off. This easily understood description of the detrimental effects of acoustic noise to hearing is a helpful comparison to the detrimental effects of image noise on the display of visual information. Both examples are random fluctuations that interfere with the communication of information.

Image noise can be defined as random variations in the OD. Other terms that have been used to describe image noise are:

- Graininess
- Granularity
- Speckle
- Salt and pepper appearance

Figure 5-4 demonstrates the appearance of image noise in a radiograph. The appearance of image noise in a mammogram is similar to a subtle and diffuse fuzziness because of the way that the noise breaks up edges in the image. The sources of noise and factors affecting noise are:

- *Image receptor:*
  - ❏ *Screen:* Nonuniformity of light emission

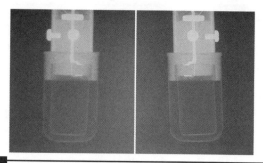

Figure 5-4 **Radiographic image noise.** The image on the right was produced with six times more radiation than the image on the left. The higher radiation dose results in lower quantum noise, which gives the appearance of a sharper image.

- ❏ *Film:* Nonuniform response to light or clumping of silver grains
- ■ *Image contrast:* High image contrast is desirable for visualizing subtle signs of pathology in a mammogram such as microcalcifications or small nodules.
  - ❏ High contrast also has the effect of increasing the amplitude of image noise.
  - ❏ Any changes that increase image contrast will also likely make image noise more apparent.
- ■ *Quantum mottle:* A component of image noise that is dependent on the number of photons that have contributed to the image. The number of photons is directly related to the radiation exposure thus patient dose. The relationship between radiation dose and image noise is, as expected, a trade-off.
  - ❏ Lower image noise, which is desirable, comes at the cost of higher radiation dose and vice versa.
  - ❏ Any action that reduces the radiation dose, such as changing from standard to extended processing, will almost certainly result in an increase in image noise.

Vignette

A few years ago, a mammography facility was using a screen-film processing combination that was at the limit of what the film manufacturer recommended. The system speed was high and, consequently, radiation doses were considerably lower than the national average. Image noise was at an acceptable level. At a certain point, the film manufacturer changed the film response slightly such that the image noise increased slightly. When the radiologist contacted me to say that the noise was too high, I determined that changes would have to be made. In my judgment, the opinion of the radiologist regarding the acceptability of image noise was the deciding factor. If the radiologist says that the noise is too high, then the noise is too high. The decision was made to remedy the unacceptable noise by switching the film processor from extended mode to standard mode. The decision was purposely made to decrease the processing efficiency, which meant that the radiation dose to all patients would be increased. The manufacturers were called in to adjust the AEC to accommodate the new processing conditions. This is a real life example of increasing the patient dose, on purpose, to reduce the image noise.

The factors that affect image noise are the same as the factors that contribute to radiation exposure, including:

- kVp
- mA
- Screen-film efficiency
- Processing speed
- OD

In nearly all cases, any changes that decrease the radiation dose will cause an increase in image noise, such as:

- Increasing the kVp
- Increasing image receptor sensitivity
- Increasing processor efficiency (e.g., extended processing)

Image Artifacts

An *artifact* can be defined as anything that is perceptible in the image but does not correspond to any anatomic or pathologic feature of the breast being imaged. Noise, as discussed in the previous section, is one example of a diffuse artifact. Artifacts that can mimic pathologic abnormalities in a mammogram or otherwise interfere with diagnosis are the most serious artifacts. Again, the interpreting radiologist has the final word as to the acceptability of specific artifacts that may be discovered. Image artifacts in a mammogram can be either plus density or minus density, sharp or diffuse, and can be caused by anything that is between the focal spot of the x-ray tube and the eye of the radiologist. The following list highlights possible contributors to image artifacts:

- X-ray tube–tube unit:
  - Window
  - Filter
  - Mirror
- Compression paddle
- Breast support
- Grid
- Patient:
  - Extraneous items that are included in the image (e.g., ear, hair or wig, skin, robe)
  - Deodorant
  - Skin lesions
  - Miscellaneous (e.g., buckshot, tattoos, knife tip)
- Image receptor:
  - Screen defects, stains, or pitting
  - *Film:* Although rare, film can come out of the box with some type of emulsion artifact, such as featherlike cracking pattern in the emulsion, tiny metal flecks on the *back* gel layer, or a scratch or buffed-appearing dark streaks.
- Darkroom:
  - Static
  - Dust or dirt:
    - Can be a big problem
    - Need hard ceiling, not acoustic tile or any other material that *sheds*
    - Follow recommended cleaning procedures, including wet wiping counter tops every day, washing floors, walls, ceiling, and power cords as needed
    - Air vents may need to be filtered
    - Air in darkroom should be at a *positive* pressure

When the door is opened, air moves out rather than moving in. If the film drop is outside the darkroom, airflow in the processor should be in the direction from developer toward fixer, and not the reverse because fixer fumes can condense on the top developer rollers, which can cause artifacts.

- Film handling:
  - Kinks or creases
  - Fingerprints
  - Pressure marks
  - Chemical deposits (e.g., hand cream)

- ■ Processor:
  - ❑ Chemistry
  - ❑ Mechanics
  - ❑ Pressure marks
  - ❑ Pick-off
  - ❑ Dirt
  - ❑ Streaks
  - ❑ Scratches
- ■ *Viewing conditions:* Illuminator dust, dirt, or marks

If an artifact appears repeatedly on images, some detective work may be required to solve the mystery, that is, to discover the source of the artifact. To review, artifacts can be caused during:

- ■ Exposure
- ■ Film handling
- ■ Processing

The following sequence of steps is suggested to track down the source of an image artifact in mammography:

- ■ Expose a pair of films, one after the other, under identical conditions, using the same film cassette.
- ■ The two films are run through the processor, one with the short length and one with the long length, parallel to the direction of motion.
- ■ Helpful hint: When tracking down artifacts, the corners should be bent on the trailing edge of the film up as it is moving into the processor, which makes it easy to know which is the leading edge and whether the emulsion was up or down.
- ■ The film pair is viewed side by side.
- ■ Artifacts that have the same orientation with respect to motion through the processor are from *processing*.
- ■ Artifacts that have the same orientation with respect to exposure are from the *imaging system*.

Artifacts from the Processor

Processor artifacts can have a number of origins, such as:

- ■ Mechanical
- ■ Chemical
- ■ Dirty wash water
- ■ Dryer too hot

Excellent artifact descriptions and troubleshooting guides with suggested remedies are available from film manufacturers. To obtain more information, contact a representative and ask for a list of available literature. The following list briefly describes common mammography processing artifacts.

- Parallel to film travel:
  - ❏ *Guide shoe marks:* (+) or (−) density, leading-trailing edges or across film, typically 1 inch apart
  - ❏ *Delay streaks:* Usually (+) density, random spacing, variable width
  - ❏ *Marks from (ribbed) entrance roller:* (+) density, typically $1/8$ inch wide
  - ❏ Scratched emulsion from crystallized chemistry on rollers
- Perpendicular to film travel:
  - ❏ *Hesitation line:* (+) density line, approximately $1 1/2$ inch behind leading edge
  - ❏ *Slap line:* Broad (+) density, approximately 2 inches from trailing edge
  - ❏ *Chatter:* (+) density, multiple, random spacing
  - ❏ *Pi lines:* Usually (+) density, 8 cm apart for 1-inch rollers
- Random orientation and location:
  - ❏ *Pick-off:* Small (−) density spots
  - ❏ *Runback:* (+) density, trailing edge, irregular edge
  - ❏ *Static:* (+) density, may appear as a lightning bolt
  - ❏ *Skiving:* Thin line of black emulsion, random locations
  - ❏ *Shadow:* White, from dust on screen
  - ❏ *Low-density smudge:* Light area from screen stain
  - ❏ *Wet pressure:* Mottled appearance, often on leading edge
  - ❏ *Dye spots:* Areas of color in the emulsion, often pinkish
  - ❏ *Surface streaks or blotches:* Uneven drying
  - ❏ *Surface dirt:* Biomass in wash
- Handling artifacts
  - ❏ *Kinks:* (+) or (−) density
  - ❏ *Fingerprint:* (+) or (−) density
  - ❏ *Deposits on film or screen:* (e.g. lipstick) usually (−) density

Clean-up film can eliminate many of these artifacts. Film designed for this purpose should be used daily to minimize artifacts.

Artifacts from the imaging system. The following considerations and sequence of steps can be used to discover the
source of an artifact produced by the imaging system:

■ *Cassette:* When the cassette is a candidate for the source
of the artifact, the first and obvious change to make is to
produce an image with another cassette. If the artifact is
gone, then the offending cassette can be inspected for
damage such as stains on the screen.

■ *Bucky mechanism or compression paddle:*
  ❏ An image can be produced with the film in the Bucky,
  but with the compression paddle removed.
  ❏ If the artifact persists, then an image can be produced
  with the cassette on top of the breast support. This
  exposure can be performed conveniently in the manual mode by using approximately one half of the mA
  that was required to produce an acceptable OD with
  the image receptor in the Bucky.

■ Grid nonuniformities and artifacts can be accentuated
by imaging the grid stationary if possible. Some grids
can be unplugged. The small Bucky can be imaged on
top of the large Bucky.
  ❏ If the artifact persists without the compression paddle and with the film-screen cassette on top of the
  Bucky, the next considerations would be the mirror,
  filter, or tube window.
  ❏ If the imaging system has a choice of filters, the next
  step would be to produce an image with another filter. (The cassette can now go back in the Bucky.)
  ❏ If artifact persists, the source of the artifact is most
  likely the mirror or the tube window. One way of
  obtaining additional information on the source of the
  artifact is to produce an image in the magnification
  mode, or with the DMR or M3000, change to the
  alternative target material.
    • Changing from the large focal spot to the small
    focal spot or from one target material to another
    moves the position of the focal spot and will
    cause a difference in magnification factor for the
    artifact. This procedure can give some clues as to

whether the artifact is in the tube assembly or in the mirror.

- The magnification is greater for artifacts in the tube window, thus they will move more in the image when the position of the x-ray source is changed.

Generally, filter and mirror artifacts can be eliminated by careful cleaning (usually by a service person). In cases of persistent artifacts that are judged significant, the only solution may be replacing a part or assembly, such as the grid, Bucky mechanism, filter, or x-ray tube. These parts or assemblies can be expensive and the decisions should be made with input from the facility, radiologist, technologist, service personnel, and physicist.

CHAPTER 6

Radiation Exposure and Patient Dose

Chapter at a glance

INTRODUCTION

As discussed in Chapter 2, x-rays are a type of *light* that can pass through soft tissues. This property can be associated with the tiny wavelength of x-rays (approximately 1 Å = 0.1 nm = 10^{-10} m). Planck's equation tells us that this small wavelength must be accompanied by high-photon energy:

$$E = \frac{hc}{\lambda}$$

> *Where:* E is photon energy
>   *h* is Planck's constant = 4.14 × 10^{-15} eVsec
>   c is the speed of light = 3 × 10^8 m/s
> $hc \simeq$ 12.4 kilo keV Å
>   λ is the wavelength

In the case of mammographic x-rays, the photon energy is approximately 18 keV. This energy is more than sufficient to dislodge electrons from their atoms, thus x-rays are referred to as *ionizing radiation*. In general, the energetic electrons ejected by ionizing radiation can produce deleterious effects, including:

- Breaking molecular bonds:
  - ❏ Can cause mutations in DNA
  - ❏ Can induce cancer in normal tissue
  - ❏ Can cause birth defects in the case of fetal exposure
- Creating free radicals such as OH (hydroxyl radical), which are chemically active and can disrupt normal cellular function
- Cross-linking (attaching) proteins
- Damaging normal tissue (high doses of radiation)
  - ❏ Skin erythema (will occur in mammography if filtration is absent)
  - ❏ Cataracts

There is, once again, a trade-off. The same radiation that is valuable for diagnosing disease has the potential (albeit small) of *causing* disease. The risk and benefit of radiation delivery must be carefully balanced. This concept is especially important for breast cancer screening, in which radiation is delivered to a large number of asymptomatic women. Before considering the risks and benefits of radiation, some basic descriptors of radiation delivery are defined.

Basic Concepts of Radiation Measurement

The x-ray beam that is delivered to a patient can be described in two ways, which will now be defined along with the units of measurement.

Radiation Exposure

Radiation exposure is a measure of the *quantity* of x-rays, the number of photons delivered, which for a typical mammographic exposure is approximately 100,000,000,000,000,000,000 (10^{20}).

- Radiation exposure can be measured directly using an exposure meter, also referred to as a dosimeter (actually a misnomer) or ion chamber.
- Exposure measurement takes advantage of the ionization that occurs as x-rays pass through air. The elec-

trons and positive ions created by the x-rays are collected in the ion chamber.

■ The traditional unit of exposure measurement is the roentgen (R) and is equal to 2.58×10^{-4} coulombs/kilograms of air. This measurement means that a certain quantity of electrical charge $1/4$ is produced when 1 kg of air (approximately 1 cubic meter) is irradiated by 1 R of x-rays.

■ The recommended unit of exposure in SI (the international system) units is coulombs/kilogram (C/kg). The conversion is 1 C/kg = 3876 R. This represents an extremely large x-ray exposure. The (R) is considerably more convenient for describing mammography radiation exposures, which are typically about 1 R.

Exposure is a useful and important x-ray measurement because it is easy to perform. Anyone with an exposure meter having a proper response to low-energy x-rays can make mammography exposure measurements that can be compared with exposure measurements made by any other investigator.

Radiation Dose

Although the measurement of exposure is convenient, it does not answer the important question, "What is the risk to the patient from this radiation?" Radiation risk and the potential for damage are related to the energy that is deposited by the x-rays as they interact with and are absorbed by tissue. Essential concepts, definitions, and methodology for calculating radiation dose are as follows:

■ Absorbed radiation dose is defined as the energy deposited per unit mass by the delivery of an x-ray exposure.

■ The traditional unit of absorbed radiation dose is the rad (**r**adiation **a**bsorbed **d**ose).

  ❑ One rad is defined as 100 ergs of energy deposited per gram (100 erg/g). An erg is a quantity of energy in an obsolete system of units (CGS).

  ❑ Typical glandular doses in mammography are less than $1/4$ rad.

■ The international system (SI) name for absorbed dose is the gray (Gy). A gray equals 100 rad (1 Gy = 100 rad).

One gray also equals 1 joule of energy deposited per kilogram of tissue.

■ Radiation dose cannot be measured directly (except with sophisticated instruments in a laboratory).

■ Patient radiation dose must be calculated.

Vignette

A rad represents an extremely small quantity of energy. Consider the following illustration: A kilogram of tissue (approximate mass of a typical breast) is reasonably represented by a liter of water. Because the density of water is 1.0, one liter of water is exactly one kilogram of water. One joule of energy deposited into a liter of water (100 rads) will raise its temperature only 4.3×10^{-4} degrees Fahrenheit. This means that about 230,000 rads would be required to raise the temperature of one liter of water 1° F. This is an extremely large radiation dose (approximately 35 times greater than the therapeutic dose that would be delivered to a patient with a tumor).

Equivalent Dose

Absorbed radiation dose (the rad and gray) are measures of the energy deposited by radiation in tissue. Equivalent dose[4,5] is a related quantity that takes into account the *biologic effects* that result from the absorbed dose.

■ The unit for equivalent dose is the rem (rad equivalent man).

■ Personnel dosimeter exposures are usually reported as the dose equivalent (rem) received.

■ The equivalent dose (in rems) is calculated by multiplying the absorbed dose (rads) by a radiation-weighting factor (w_R) for the radiation being used. W_R was formerly called the quality factor (Q).

■ The unit of equivalent dose is also 1 joule per kilogram. The SI name for equivalent dose is the sievert (Sv).

■ 1 sievert (Sv) = 100 rem

■ The weighting factor (w_R) for x-rays is 1, which means that for mammography, *1 rad is also 1 rem*. 1 rad = 1 rem and 1 Gy = 1 Sv.

Effective Dose

The effective dose[4,5] is a dose-reporting scheme that can be used to calculate the overall effect when the whole body is not irradiated or when more than one tissue or organ is irradiated, as with whole-body irradiation.

- Tissue-weighting factors are assigned to specific tissues or organs for total body irradiation. The tissue weighting factors (w_T) add up to 1.0.
- The tissue-weighting factor for breast is 0.05.
- Therefore an equivalent dose of 1 rem to the breast gives an effective dose of 0.05 × 1000 mrem = 50 mrem.
- Therefore a breast dose of 1 rem is thought to have the same effect as a whole-body dose of 50 mrem.

Mean Glandular Dose

Currently, mammography is the only radiographic procedure for which there is universal agreement on how radiation dose should be calculated and reported. Dose specification and reporting in mammography should always be in terms of mean glandular dose[6] (D_g).

- Mean glandular dose is the same as *average glandular dose.*
- Calculated using the following scheme:
  - ❏ Radiation *exposure* to the breast (R) is multiplied by:
  - ❏ An *exposure-to-dose conversion factor* that depends on:
    - Half-value layer (effective x-ray beam energy)
    - Breast thickness
    - Other factors to a lesser extent, including filter and anode material, breast tissue type, and kilovolts peak (kVp).
  - ❏ Tables have been published that can be used to determine the roentgen-to-rad conversion factor.[7]

Calculating Mean Glandular Dose

If there is ever a need or desire to determine a specific patient radiation dose delivered in a mammography examination, the following equation can be used to calculate the mean glandular dose for a particular radiation exposure.[8]

$$D_g = (R) \times (HVL) \times (1/T) \times 2.1$$

Where: D_g is the absorbed dose in millirads (mrad)
E is the exposure in milliroentgens (mR)
HVL is the half-value layer (in mm) of aluminum
T is the breast thickness (in cm)

The results given by this equation agree within 2% to 3% to the values reported by the tables previously referenced for all the target-filter-kVp combinations commonly used for mammography.

This equation has been implemented in a calculating device (Figure 6-1).[9] To use the device, the wheel is turned until the set kVp is aligned with the mAs reported for the exposure. The dose is then read directly adjacent to the breast thickness for the appropriate tissue composition: dense, fatty, or average.

Typical Doses

Radiation technologists and radiologists should have enough understanding of radiation physics and effects to discuss the possible risks associated with diagnostic exposures with their patients. A few radiation facts should be understood by all radiation workers:

- The average effective dose from background radiation in the United States is about 350 mrem (3.5 mSv) per year.[10]
- 300 mrem of the background is referred to as annual *natural background radiation*.
    - ❏ Approximately 200 mrem is effective dose to the bronchial epithelium from radon gas inhalation.
    - ❏ Approximately 100 mrem is from cosmic, other terrestrial, and internal sources (which are all slightly radioactive).

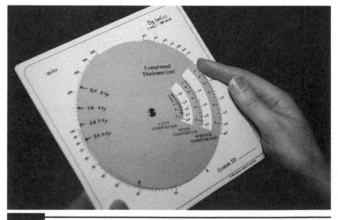

Figure 6-1 A circular slide rule device is used for a quick and simple calculation of patient average glandular dose in mammography.

- ❏ An additional estimated 50 mrem comes from man-made sources, which include medical, nuclear medicine, consumer products, and other sources.
- The annual dose limit for occupational workers, which includes mammography technologists, is *5 rem* (5000 mrem, 50 mSv). This limit applies to whole body exposure, it was formerly known as the maximum permissible dose (MPD) for occupational workers.[4]
- There is no dose limit for patients (except mammography), but every radiation delivery must be prescribed by a physician.

A couple of other radiation facts that are particularly relevant to mammography, and that should be known by all mammography technicians are:

- The maximum mean glandular dose that can be delivered to a phantom approved by the U. S. Food and Drug Administration (FDA) that simulates a standard breast is limited by federal law to *300 mrad* (3 mGy).[11]
  - ❏ This hypothetical *standard breast* is loosely represented by the American College of Radiology (ACR) accreditation phantom. However, between the 1992 and the 1994 mammography quality control manuals, the ACR changed the breast thickness represented by the phantom from 4.5 to 4.2 cm. (This change caused a 7% *overnight* increase in facility mean glandular dose for identical radiation exposures to that phantom.)
  - ❏ This same dose limit is recommended by the American College of Radiology.[7]
  - ❏ Some states have tightened this limit to 200 mrad.
- The national average of the mean glandular dose measured by the FDA inspectors for exposures of the mammography accreditation phantom in 1997 was 1.60 mGy (160 mrad).[12] This figure is higher than the national average in 1992 of 1.49. The increase is most likely a result of an increase in the average OD of mammograms over the same period, from 1.18 to 1.52 OD.[12]
- Therefore the national average dose in 1997, as measured with the accreditation phantom, was approximately 50% of the maximal permissible mammography dose.

- Before moving on to consider the risks and benefits of mammography, the following should be considered:
  - ❑ The effective dose from a typical screening mammography examination is $E = 200$ mrad $\times$ 2 exposures $\times$ ($w_T = 0.05$) $= 20$ mrem.

The typical effective dose for a screening mammography examination is less than 3 weeks of background dose.

  - ❑ The effective dose from a screening mammography examination is approximately 0.5% of the annual dose limit for the technologist performing the examination. In fact, if a mammography technologist had a screening mammography study every month for a year, she would still be under her annual effective dose limit (whole body and breast) as an occupational worker.

PUTTING RADIATION DOSE IN PERSPECTIVE

Life is full of risks. Everyday, people voluntarily submit themselves to risks that are much greater than the risks associated with diagnostic level radiation doses (e.g., driving a car, smoking cigarettes, being overweight). What is known about the health risks of radiation?

Health Risks of Radiation

- High doses of radiation are known to be detrimental to health.
  - ❑ A single whole-body dose of 500 rads gives a 50-50 chance of death.
  - ❑ 200 rads to the skin will cause radiation burns.
  - ❑ 200 to 300 rads to the lens of the eyes will likely cause a cataract.
- There are no *proven* detrimental effects from diagnostic doses of x-rays (less than a few rads), although there is a continuing debate on this subject.
- Published risks for diagnostic doses are hypothetical and are calculated based on the known effects of large radiation exposures using the most conservative (linear; no threshold) hypothesis for extrapolation.

- A typical analysis of the hypothetical risk of inducing a fatal cancer from undergoing mammography can be as follows:
  - ❏ A conservative risk of inducing a fatal cancer with radiation is taken to be 4×10^{-4} per rem,[4] which means that 1 out of 2500 persons receiving 1 rem of (whole-body) dose may die from a cancer that was caused by the radiation.
  - ❏ The effective dose from a screening mammography examination was calculated to be typically 20 mrem.
  - ❏ This radiation level produces a risk of fatal cancer induction for screening mammography of approximately 20 mrem $\times$ (4×10^{-4} per rem) = 8×10^{-6} (8 per million).
  - ❏ If an individual has screening mammography every year for 40 years, then the risk of inducing a fatal cancer becomes approximately $8 \times 10^{-6} \times 40$ or approximately 3×10^{-4} (3 per 10,000).

Putting It All Together

Screening mammography for an individual for 40 years has a potential to induce a fatal cancer in approximately 3 out of 10,000 individuals. However, in these same 10,000 women, by age 80, there may be, for example, 1000 cases of breast cancer. If only half of the cancers can be detected and treated (including any that may have been induced), about 500 cancer deaths may be prevented by screening mammography.

This simplistic presentation involves some assumptions and uncertainties, but it makes the point that should be understood: *the risks associated with good screening mammography, although not zero, are low and are much less than the risks of undetected cancer.*

Several steps can be taken to decrease the radiation dose delivered to the population by mammography, the most obvious being to quit mammography. However, currently in the United States, there is a consensus that the benefits of annual screening mammography beginning at age 40 clearly outweigh the risks. The current priority for mammography is early and accurate detection of breast cancer.

CHAPTER 7

Mammography Quality Control

Chapter at a glance

INTRODUCTION

Quality control and quality assurance are terms that describe a program for the improvement and maintenance of quality in radiology. Let us begin with some definitions taken from Report 99 of the National Council on Radiation Protection and Measurements.[13]

Definitions

■ *Quality control* is a series of distinct technical procedures that ensure the production of a satisfactory product. Its aim is to provide quality that is not only satisfactory and diagnostic, but also dependable and economic.

■ *Quality assurance* is an all-encompassing program, including quality control, that extends to administrative, educational, and preventative maintenance methods and includes a continuing evaluation of the adequacy and effectiveness of the overall imaging program, with a view to initiating corrective measures when necessary.

Benefits

The traditional justification and motivation for providing quality control has been the *3 Ds:*

- Diagnosis
- Dose
- Dollars

Quality control (QC) and quality assurance (QA) can help achieve the desired goal of producing consistently high-quality images with the minimal radiation dose necessary to achieve the desired image quality. In nearly every case, the radiation dose can easily be reduced for any given radiologic examination at the expense of reduced image quality. However, patients are irradiated because of the potentially significant benefits to them provided by the examination. Technicians should always strive to achieve a maximal image–quality-to-dose ratio (high image quality or low radiation dose). This principle of using the lowest dose consistent with the requirements of the diagnostic examination is often expressed using the acronym ALARA, which means *as low as reasonably achievable.*

The potential benefits of QC-QA are well known. However, there are also costs associated with the performance of QC-QA that include film, technologist time, equipment, and frustration, to mention a few. To maximize the benefit to cost ratio, the costs should be minimized.

- What technical factors should be tested?
- How often should these factors be tested?

To answer these questions, two additional questions should be asked:

- How does this technical factor affect image quality?
- How likely is image quality to change?

MAMMOGRAPHY ACCREDITATION PROGRAM: HISTORICAL BACKGROUND

For better or for worse, the decisions regarding what to test and how often, have been made for us by the American College of Radiology (ACR) as recommended in their mammography accreditation program (MAP).[7] The voluntary ACR and mandatory federal programs represent a significant change for radiology. Mammography is the first modality where the *practice* of radiology is regulated.

A short history of this development is worth considering:

■ *1987:* ACR initiates a voluntary accreditation program for mammography.

■ *October 27, 1992:* President George Bush signed the Mammography Quality Standards Act (MQSA) to take effect October 1, 1994.

■ *1992:* The first ACR Mammography Quality Control Manual is published.

■ *Interim regulations were published in the Federal Register on December 23, 1993:* These regulations required federal certification of all mammography facilities as of October 1, 1994. The ACR QC program was adopted by reference as the MQSA QC program.

■ *1994:* The second ACR Mammography Quality Control Manual is published.

■ *The final MQSA regulations were published on October 28, 1997 and took effect April 29, 1999:* These regulations include a *required* QC program that is similar but not identical to the ACR program. The specifications of the ACR QC program became *recommendations;* they are not required for FDA certification.

■ *September 25, 1998:* Congress passed the MQSA Reauthorization Act, which became effective on April 28,1999 and extended the FDA authority to carry out the regulations.

■ *1999:* The ACR Mammography Quality Control Manual, modified to compliment MQSA requirements for QC, was published.

Compliance with all MQSA requirements is necessary to obtain FDA certification of mammography facilities. This certification is required to practice mammography legally in the United States.

■ ACR (or state) accreditation has been retained as part of MQSA to ensure competent evaluation of the clinical mammography program, including clinical image quality.

■ The QC program for mammography has been standardized and is essentially codified in the final MQSA regulations.

■ The FDA has published four guidance documents to answer questions about compliance with the regulations (late-year 2000).

- All FDA MQSA materials, including the regulation, guidance documents, facility inspection statistics, and the MQSA newsletter, *Mammography Matters*, are retrievable from their web site at www.fda.gov/cdrh/dmqrp.html. MQSA hotline is (800) 838-7715.
- The current QC procedures recommended by the ACR are specified in their 1999 Quality Control Manual.[6]
- Adherence with ACR procedures will satisfy the FDA requirements for certification pertaining to QC.
- Compliance with ACR recommendations, when they are stricter than MQSA, is optional. These include (mid-year 2000):
  - ❏ X-ray field size compared with the image receptor
  - ❏ Tolerance for OD variation in automatic exposure control (AEC) tests
  - ❏ Half-value layer (HVL) limits
  - ❏ Radiation output rate
  - ❏ Illuminator brightness
- Individual states, as accrediting bodies or as part of their own radiation control program, can mandate compliance with requirements that are more strict than MQSA.
- The FDA is considering authorizing states to be the certifying agency *and* the accreditation body for mammography facilities in that state.

MAMMOGRAPHY QUALITY STANDARDS ACT

Because of the importance of MQSA and the difficulty experienced by many individuals attempting to wade through the Federal Register, a comprehensive outline and summary of the final regulations, is presented here. The original numbering is retained to facilitate using this summary with the actual regulation published in the *Federal Register;* volume 62, number 208, pages 55,976–55,994 (excluding comments). The material contained in 900.12 entitled, *Quality Standards* is most relevant to mammography facilities and personnel and is presented in an expanded format. If specific compliance questions arise, the original regulation and compliance documents should be consulted, or the FDA can be contacted directly by phone ([800] 838-7715), fax ([301] 986-8015), or through the FDA web site at www.fda.gov/cdrh/dmqrp.html.

▌Final MQSA Regulations

PART 900—Mammography—index

900.12 Quality Standards—outline and summary

(a) Personnel

1. Interpreting physicians
    (i) *initial qualifications*
        (A) *be licensed to practice medicine in a state*
        (B) *(1) be certified by an FDA approved specialty board -or-*
            (2) have 3 months formal training in mammogram interpretation

      (C) have ≥ 60 hours of education in mammography

      (D) have read ≥ 240 mammographic exams in
          previous 6 months

  (ii) continuing experience and education

      (A) read ≥ 960 mammographic exams in any
          2-year period

      (B) have 15 credits of continuing education in any
          3 year period

  (iii) exemptions

  (iv) reestablishing qualifications

2. Radiologic technologist

  (i) general

      (A) have a general license in a state –or–

      (B) have a general certificate from FDA approved
          certifying body

  (ii) mammographic requirements
     must have qualified as mammographic technologist
     prior to April 28,1999 -or-
     have completed 40 contact hours of mammographic
     training including:

      (A) breast anatomy and physiology, positioning,
          compression, QC/QA and imaging patients with
          implants

      (B) performance of at least 25 exams under
          qualified direct supervision

      (C) have at least 8 hours training in each modality
          used (e.g., screen-film)

  (iii) continuing education (CE)

      (A) 15 CEU per 3 year period following initial
          qualification, and thereafter

      (B) teaching hours can be counted once only

      (C) at least 6 hours of CE devoted to each modality
          used

      (D) if qualification lapses—CE must be obtained to
          meet (A) and (C)

      (E) 8 hours of CE in any new modality prior to use

  (iv) continuing experience

      (A) perform at least 200 exams per 2 year period
          following initial qualification, and thereafter

      (B) if qualification lapses—at least 25 supervised
          exams must be performed

3. Medical physicist (not expanded here)
4. Retention of personnel records
   records documenting the qualification of all personnel must be kept, records for departed individuals must be kept until next MQSA inspection

(b) Equipment

1. Prohibited equipment
   general purpose equipment shall not be used for mammography
2. General
   mammography must be performed with specifically designed and FDA compliant equipment
3. Motion of tube-image receptor assembly
   (i) *assembly can be fixed solidly in any orientation for which it is designed to work*
   (ii) *mechanism fixing orientation shall not release in case of power failure*
4. Image receptor sizes
   (i) *screen-film receptors of 18 $\times$ 24 and 24 $\times$ 30 cm must be provided*
   (ii) *Bucky grids must be provided for each screen-film image receptor*
   (iii) *grid mechanism must be removable for magnification imaging*
5. Beam limitation and light fields
   (i) *(requirement removed by amendment 4/7/99)*
   (ii) *average light field illumination must be > 160 lux (15 fc)*
6. Magnification
   (i) *diagnostic systems must have capability for radiographic magnification*
   (ii) *magnification between 1.4 and 2.0 must be provided*
7. Focal spot selection
   (i) *if two focal spots are offered, the one chosen must be displayed prior to exposure*
   (ii) *if multiple targets are provided, the one chosen must be displayed prior to exposure*
   (iii) *if the system chooses the technique, it must be displayed post-exposure*

8. Compression

   all systems must provide compression

   (i) Effective **October 28, 2002** systems shall provide:

     (A) initial "hands-free" power drive from both sides of patient

     (B) fine adjustment available from both sides of patient

   (ii) compression paddle:

     (A) a compression paddle corresponding to each image receptor must be provided

     (B) unless designed to operate differently, the compression paddle must be flat and parallel to the breast support (within 1 cm)

     (C) other equipment must meet manufacturer's design specifications

     (D) chest wall edge must be straight and parallel to image receptor

     (E) chest wall edge may be bent upward but must not appear on image

9. Technique factor selection and display

   (i) manual selection of mA & time or mAs must be provided

   (ii) selected kVp and mAs must be displayed pre-exposure (for non-AEC)

   (iii) for AEC operation, kVp and mAs shall be displayed post-exposure

10. Automatic exposure control

   (i) screen-film systems shall provide AEC for all operating modes

   (ii) flexible detector positioning must be provided

     (A) size and position choices must be indicated on compression paddle

     (B) selected position must be clearly indicated

   (iii) optical density compensation shall be provided (+/− adjustment)

11. X-ray film

   film used shall be designated appropriate for mammography

12. Intensifying screens

   screens used shall be designated by the manufacturer as appropriate for mammography and compatible with the film used

13. Film processing solutions
    chemistry must provide the performance level specified by film manufacturer

14. Lighting
    a "hot light" shall be provided to the interpreting physician

15. Film masking devices
    devices to limit the illuminated area to less than or equal to the exposed area must be provided

(c) Medical records and mammography reports

1. report must contain:
   (i) *patient name and ID*
   (ii) *examination date*
   (iii) *name of interpreting physician*
   (iv) *overall final assessment using approved terminology (negative, benign, prob. benign, suspicious, highly suggestive of malignancy) if indeterminate— "incomplete-need additional images"*
   (v) *recommendations for next action to be taken (if any)*

2. results (written) must be communicated to patient (non-negative ASAP)
   (i) *ASAP but not more than 30 days (patients without personal physician get report with summary)*
   (ii) *patients without own physician shall be referred to one when required*

3. communication with health care providers
   (i) *written report ASAP but within 30 days*
   (ii) *for non-negative assessments ASAP to primary physician or designee*

4. record-keeping; facilities performing mammography exams shall:
   (i) *keep films at least 5 years (10 if patient doesn't return) unless requested by patient*
   (ii) *if requested by or on behalf of patient, transfer original films*
   (iii) *any fee charged for transfer shall not exceed costs*

5. each mammogram shall have the following identification:
   (i) *name and ID of patient*

      (ii)   *date of exam*

      (iii) *view and laterality following recommendations of accrediting body*

      (iv) *facility name and address*

      (v)   *technologist identification*

      (vi) *mammography unit ID*

(d) Quality assurance—general

1. Responsible individuals

    (i)   *lead interpreting physician—overall responsibility for QA program*

    (ii) *interpreting physicians—support corrective actions, medical audit*

    (iii) *medical physicist—annual survey and equipment evaluations*

    (iv) *QC technologist—do or supervise all QA duties not otherwise assigned*

2. Quality assurance records (personnel, imaging techniques, QC, safety etc.); keep records longest of next MQSA inspection or until test repeated 2 times

(e) Quality assurance—equipment

1. Daily quality control tests
processor control

    (i)   *B + F within + 0.03 OD*

    (ii) *MD + 0.15 OD*

    (iii) *DD + 0.15 OD*

2. Weekly quality control tests
phantom (for screen-film imaging)

    (i)   *OD > 1.20*

    (ii) *OD + 0.20*

    (iii) *image quality satisfying accreditation body requirements*

    (iv) *DD + 0.05 OD*

3. Quarterly quality control tests

    (i)   *fixer retention $\leq 5\mu$ g/cm^2*

    (ii) *repeat analysis—variation $\leq 2\%$ total films*

4. Semiannual quality control tests

    (i)   *darkroom fog— < 0.05 OD*

(ii) *screen-film contact*

(iii) *compression*

    (A) *force* > 111 N (25 lb)

    (B) **Oct. 28, 2002:** *max. initial force between 111-209 N (25-47 lb)*

5. Annual quality control tests

  (i) *AEC*

    (A) *OD within ± 0.30 mean for 2-6 cm (or correct with technique chart)*

    (B) **Oct. 28, 2002:** *OD within ± 0.15 for 2-6 cm*

    (C) *OD in image center ≥ 1.20*

  (ii) *kVp*

    (A) *accurate within 5% of indicated value at:*

      (1) *lowest measurable clinical kVp*

      (2) *most commonly used kVp*

      (3) *highest available clinical kVp*

    (B) *CV of reproducibility ≤ 0.02 at most commonly used kVp*

  (iii) *focal spot*

    system resolution or size until Oct. 28, 2002; resolution only, thereafter

    (A) *system resolution*

      (1) *≥ 11 lp/mm (length) and ≥ 13 lp/mm (width)*

      (2) *resolution pattern centered, 4.5 cm above breast support*

      (3) *each target tested separately*

      (4) *test at most commonly used SID*

      (5) *typical kVp used in AEC mode (screen-film in Bucky)*

    (B) *focal spot size: 0.1 − 0.2mm + 50% (l&w), > 0.2mm + 50%w + 115% l*

  (iv) *HVL − HVL > (kVp/100)*

  (v) *exposure reproducibility—CV for air kerma and mAs < 0.05*

  (vi) *dosimetry—mean glandular dose for accepted phantom, × mGy (300 mrad)*

  (vii) *x-ray/light field/compression paddle alignment*

    (A) *x-ray field must extend beyond chest wall edge of image receptor, cannot be more than 2% SID*

    beyond any edge of the image receptor
    (amended 4/7/99)
- (B) total x-ray/light misalignment (l or w) < 2%
    SID
- (C) chest wall edge of compression paddle within
    1% SID beyond image receptor (at standard
    thickness), but not visible in image
    (viii) screen speed uniformity (and artifacts)—(max. OD
    − min. OD) ≤ 0.03
    (ix) artifacts—test all cassettes, grids, focal spots,
    target/filter combinations
    (x) radiation output
    (A) output ≥ 513 mR/sec at 28 kVp, standard
        mode, 4.5 cm above breast support with paddle
        in beam; 800 mR/sec after **Oct. 28, 2002**
    (B) total output must be delivered in a 3 second (or
        shorter) exposure
    (xi) if automatic decompression is provided, there must be
    (A) an override capability
    (B) a continuous display of override status
    (C) a manual emergency release
6. Quality control tests—other modalities (digital)
   for other than screen-film systems—follow image
   receptor manufacturer's recommendations, but mean
   glandular dose must always be less than 300 mrad.
7. Mobile units
   system must meet (e)(1) through (e)(6) listed here;
   before imaging patients at any location, adequacy of
   image quality must be established
8. Use of test results
   (i) after performing tests (e)(1)—(e)(7), the results
       shall be compared to allowable deviations in
       performance to see if action is required
   (ii) if any test is outside of acceptable limits—corrective
       action will be taken
   (A) before clinical images are taken or processed
       (for some problems)
   (B) within 30 days of the test (for other specified
       problems)

9. Surveys
    (i) *annual survey by a qualified medical physicist—at least (e)(5) & (e)(6)*
    (ii) *physics survey will incorporate an evaluation of the QA program including any required corrective actions taken*
    (iii) *the physicist shall provide a report of the annual survey including any recommendations for improvement*
    (iv) *survey report shall be sent within 30 days of the survey*
    (v) *survey report shall be dated and signed by the medical physicist*
10. Mammography equipment evaluations (Medical Physicist)
    additional evaluations of equipment following installation, modification or repair of major components to assure compliance with standards 900.12 (b) and (e). Problems must be corrected before equipment use.
11. Facility cleanliness
    (i) *procedure required for cleaning darkroom, screens and veiwboxes*
    (ii) *performance of required protocols must be documented*
12. Calibration of air kerma measuring instruments (ion chambers)
    calibration must occur at least once per 2 years to 6% accuracy, traceable to a national standard in the mammography energy range
13. Infection control
    establish and follow systematic cleaning and disinfecting of imaging equipment after contact with potentially infectious materials, system must specify procedures and documentation that:
    (i) *comply with all Federal, State and local regulations*
    (ii) *comply with equipment manufacturer recommendations –or-*
    (iii) *comply with generally accepted procedures*

(f) **Quality assurance—mammography medical outcomes audit**
  1. all facilities shall collect and review outcome data including follow-up and correlation with pathology for all positive mammographic studies and retrospective follow-up and study of films for any cancer discovered subsequent to the exam
  2. analysis of data shall occur at least every 12 months beginning with 4/28/99
  3. at least one interpreting physician shall have the responsibility for the annual outcome audit review, including notification, follow-up action and documentation

(g) **Procedure and techniques for mammography of patients with breast implants**
  1. there shall be a procedure to inquire of all patients whether they have implants
  2. unless there is reason not to, implant patients shall have special views

(h) **Consumer complaint mechanism—each facility shall:**
  1. have a written and documented system for collecting and resolving complaints
  2. keep a record of all serious complaints for 3 years
  3. give patients directions for filing complaints with accreditation body if necessary
  4. report unresolved serious complaints to accreditation body per it's policy

(i) **Clinical image quality**
   clinical image quality must comply with standards of the accreditation body

(j) **Additional mammography review and patient notification**
  1. FDA can order additional review if they believe it's required
  2. if FDA deems it necessary, patients will be notified of possible health risk

Summary of Identified Individuals and Responsibilities

All individuals involved in the QA program must be qualified and given adequate time to perform the assigned tasks.

■ Lead interpreting physician:

❏ *MQSA*: Responsible for ensuring that all MQSA requirements for the QA program are met, including assessing the adequacy of the qualifications of all personnel

❏ *ACR*:
  - *Ensure technologist training and continuing education compliance*
  - *Provide technologist orientation program*
  - *Ensure that effective QC is being performed (motivation, oversight, and direction)*
  - *Select the primary QC technologist*
  - *Ensure availability of appropriate QC test equipment*
  - *Ensure that adequate time is available for QC testing and documentation*
  - *Provide frequent and consistent feedback to technologists about image quality*
  - *Select a qualified medical physicist*
  - *Review QC records at least quarterly, physicist report at least annually*
  - *Perform or supervise a radiation safety program*
  - *Ensure that all QC, employee qualifications, mammography technique and procedures, radiation safety, and infection control records are current and properly maintained in the QC procedures manual*
  - *Thoroughly understand key QC test procedures, especially film processing and image viewing conditions*

■ Interpreting physicians:

❏ *MQSA*:
  - Follow procedures for corrective action if images are of poor quality
  - Participate in the medical outcomes audit

❏ *ACR*:
  - *Follow procedures for corrective action if they judge images to be of poor quality*
  - *To participate in the medical outcomes audit*
  - *Provide required documentation of qualifications*
  - *Perform ongoing QA assessment of the quality of mammogram interpretation*

- Medical physicist:
  - ❑ *MQSA:*
    - Oversee equipment QA program
    - Perform annual survey and issue a detailed report
    - Perform equipment evaluations with associated report, when required
  - ❑ *ACR:*
    - *Perform annual survey including image quality, patient dose, and operator safety*
    - *Review QC testing performed by the on-sight technologist*
    - *Provide recommendations for improvement, if necessary*
    - *Perform appropriate tests following equipment installation or major service*
- Quality control technologist:
  - ❑ *MQSA:* responsible—either to perform or to supervise—all QA tasks not assigned to the lead interpreting physician or physicist
  - ❑ *ACR:*
    - *Ensure that patient care and image quality meet facility standards*
    - *Perform required QC testing at required intervals*

OBSERVATIONS, TIPS, AND RECOMMENDATIONS

Indeed, there is a new challenge in mammography, that of keeping up and complying with regulatory requirements! The following are a few tips for success:

- Visit the MQSA web site regularly to see what is new.
- Contact the FDA or ACR directly if questions arise.
- Section 900.2 contains a list of definitions that may be helpful.
- Document in writing those who are the *responsible* individuals.
  - ❑ Make sure that everyone knows their responsibilities.
  - ❑ Make the physicist a member of the team (he or she should provide a way to contact him or her, if necessary).
- Document procedures.
  - ❑ Refer to ACR manual for QC procedures (easiest way to comply with MQSA requirements).
  - ❑ Do not forget infection control (e)(13) and patient complaints (h).

- Document all relevant actions:
  - ❑ Changes in procedure or personnel
  - ❑ Problems encountered and any remedial action taken
  - ❑ Repairs performed, including any recommended repairs by the physicist
  - ❑ Required retesting by physicist or service personnel
- Section 900.12(e)(10) describes the equipment evaluation:
  - ❑ A new physicist survey
  - ❑ Required *before* imaging patients when a significant change is made involving equipment and processors.
  - ❑ *Ask a physicist if there is any question about the need for testing.*
- Sections 900.12(e)(1)-(4) define the technologist QC tests.
  - ❑ Be aware of required intervals (weekly does not mean on the same day each week).
  - ❑ Be aware of the allowed variation.
  - ❑ Record required results.
  - ❑ Keep films as required.
- Section 900.12(e)(5) defines the QC tests required of the physicist for screen-film mammography and the QC tests that must be included in the report.
  - ❑ Review the report for valuable information, in particular:
  - ❑ Noncompliance problems requiring repair (30 days).
  - ❑ Recommendations for improving quality.
  - ❑ Any artifacts identified.
  - ❑ Radiation dose and image quality.
  - ❑ AEC: Overall optical density and compensation step sizes.

Compliance efforts can be overwhelming at times, but the patient and the real purpose of mammography can never be forgotten. Even if mammographic technicians are not appreciated, *they are important!*

References

1. Ries L, Kosary C, Hankey B, Miller B, Edwards B. *SEER cancer statistics review,* Bethesda MD: National Cancer Institute, 1999.

2. Tucker DM, Barnes GT, Wu X. Molybdenum target x-ray spectra: a semiempiric model. *Med Phys* 1991;18:402–407.

3. Jacobson DR. Appropriate use of anode/filter combinations in mammography. *Med Phys* 1996;23(6):1117.

4. ICRP Publication 60. *Recommendations of the ICRP.* International Commission on Radiation Protection. Elmsford, NY: Pergamon, 1991.

5. NCRP Report 116. *Limitation of exposure to ionizing radiation.* Bethesda, MD: National Council on Radiation Protection and Measurements, 1993.

6. NCRP Report 85. *Mammography—a user's guide.* Bethesda, MD: National Council on Radiation Protection and Measurements, 1986.

7. American College of Radiology. *Mammography quality control manual.* Reston VA: American College of Radiology, 1999.

8. Jacobson DR. Radiographic exposure calculator and mammographic dose calculator. *Radiology* 1992;182:578–580.

9. Radiological Diagnostic Products, Inc., Waukesha, WI 53187.

10. NCRP Report 93. *Ionizing radiation exposure of the population of the United States.* Bethesda, MD: National Council on Radiation Protection and Measurements, 1987.

11. 21CFR 900.12(e)(5)(vi). *Federal Register* 1997;62(208):55990.

12. Suleiman OH, Spelic DC, McCrohan JL, Symonds GR, Houn F. Mammography in the 1990s: the United States and Canada. *Radiology* 1999;210:345–351.

13. NCRP Report 99. *Quality assurance for diagnostic imaging equipment.* Bethesda, MD: National Council on Radiation Protection and Measurements, 1988.

Index